Minor Tooth Movement in the Growing Child

M. MICHAEL COHEN, Sr., D.M.D.

Lecturer on Oral Pathology, Harvard School of Dental Medicine, Boston; Director of Dental Services, Lakeville Hospital, Lakeville, Massachusetts; Senior Associate Dental Department, Children's Hospital Medical Center, Boston, Massachusetts; Consultant in Pediatric Dentistry, Developmental Evaluation Clinic, Children's Hospital Medical Center, Boston; Consultant in Oral Pathology and Pediatric Dentistry, Eunice Kennedy Shriver Center and The Walter E. Fernald State School, Waltham, Massachusetts; Consultant in Oral Pathology and Pediatric Dentistry, Southbury Training School, Southbury, Connecticut.

With contributions by
JOHN R. ORR, Jr., D.M.D.
and
GERALD BORELL, A.B., D.D.S., F.A.C.D.

1977   W. B. SAUNDERS COMPANY / Philadelphia / London / Toronto

W. B. Saunders Company: West Washington Square
                           Philadelphia, PA   19105

                           1 St. Anne's Road
                           Eastbourne, East Sussex BN21 3UN, England

                           833 Oxford Street
                           Toronto, Ontario M8Z 5T9, Canada

Library of Congress Cataloging in Publication Data

Cohen, Meyer Michael,
    Minor tooth movement in the growing child.

    Includes index.
    1. Malocclusion.   2. Pedodontia.   3. Orthodontia. I. Orr, John R., joint author.   II. Borell,
Gerald, joint author.   III. Title. [DNLM: 1. Malocclusion—In infancy and childhood.   2. Tooth
movement, Minor—In infancy and childhood WU440 C678m]
RK523.C63   617.6′43   76–8570
ISBN   0-7216-2632-7

Minor Tooth Movement in the Growing Child   ISBN   0-7216-2632-7

Last digit is the print number: 9   8   7   6   5   4   3   2   1

TO THE YOUNGER GENERATION

My Grandchildren

A. M. C. ♂   J. D. C. ♂   J. M. C. ♀

and

H. S. P.   *Two Dear Young Friends*   L. B. P.
♀   ♀

COLLABORATORS

JOHN R. ORR, JR., D.M.D.
Fellow, Academy of General Dentistry
Diplomate, International Board of Orthodontics
Member, European Orthodontic Society

GERALD BORELL, A.B., D.D.S., F.A.C.D.
Associate Professor, Department of Orthodontics,
New York College of Dentistry

FOREWORD

During the next decade the evolution that is now under way in the delivery of health services will become intensified substantially, and irreversible changes will occur. At present there is a gap between medical knowledge and the delivery of health services to a significant majority of the population in the United States. It has become apparent that the present system of health care is inefficient in being inaccessible and costly to a large segment of the population.

In order to meet the health needs of this country it is quite conceivable that there will be a national health insurance and financing system based on the principles of our social security trust fund operations. The federal government, together with the citizens and health managers (formerly public health officers), will be the major participants in quality control activities, including the private practice of medicine and dentistry.

Programs of preventive care and education will gain in acceptance. In dentistry it will become mandatory for the dental practitioner to participate in the prevention of occlusal disharmonies.

This volume will deal with the recognition and treatment of minor occlusal disharmonies in the primary and early mixed dentition in order to prevent major occlusal disharmonies. The text will discuss, illustrate and differentiate between minor and major occlusal disharmonies. Casts of the occlusal relationships and intraoral Panorex and cephalometric roentgenograms are essential for establishing a diagnosis and for differentiating between a major and a minor occlusal disharmony. When an occlusal disharmony is present the parent should always be informed, and treatment should be instituted early to prevent an exacerbation of the condition.

The pediatric dentist and dental practitioner who has had training in orthodontics is capable of providing the necessary orthodontic treatment for the young child; those who have not had sufficient training and experience in orthodontics for the child with a primary or early mixed dentition occlusal disharmony should refer the patient to an orthodontist.

Together, the general practitioner, the pedodontist and the orthodontist can provide for the children of this country a pleasing appearance and a satisfactory occlusal relationship, which is an essential factor for the maintenance of a healthy dentition.

M. Michael Cohen, Sr.

PREFACE

In 1907, one year before Victor Vasarely* was born, Edward H. Angle published the seventh edition of *Treatment of Malocclusion of the Teeth*. The Angle classification of malocclusion became firmly established as a method for assessing occlusal relationships. This classification was based on a fixed relationship of the permanent maxillary first molars, in which the mandibular arch occupies either a neutral, a Class I relationship, a distal Class II relationship, or a mesial Class III relationship to the maxillary arch. When casts of the dentition are made and articulated, the occlusal relationship is determined with the teeth in centric relationship.

Angle based his concept on the perceptual ability of the dentist using plaster casts. Angle has given the dental profession a method of employing dental casts in which minor occlusal disharmonies may be observed and treated in the primary, mixed and permanent dentitions. This book will emphasize the importance of careful clinical examination and the use of dental casts as well as roentgenograms in observing early minor occlusal disharmonies. Unlike the case with orthodontic treatment, it is not necessary to have a profound knowledge of growth and development of the dentofacial complex to treat and correct minor occlusal disharmonies. Any graduate of a modern dental school is capable of detecting minor occlusal disharmonies provided that he looks as carefully for these minor deviations as he does for cavities and periodontal disease. The growth and development of the dentofacial complex is challenging and provides the practicing dentist with an opportunity to indulge in other than routine dental care. He will observe early major occlusal disharmonies in the early primary and mixed dentitions and treat them if he has had orthodontic training and experience; otherwise major occlusal disharmonies should be referred to the orthodontist for observation and treatment. Allowing the dentofacial complex to go untreated until the adolescent and postadolescent periods makes treatment more difficult and more expensive, and a successful result may never be achieved. When the orthodontist or dental

---

*Victor Vasarely, born in Pecs, Hungary, in 1908, has as an artist condensed his art into a convenient formula. Vasarely's world of forms should be universally intelligible since he continually strives to set free those forms that can be experienced spontaneously. This famous Hungarian artist bases the message and effect of his art on the human perceptual ability that lies beyond experience of history, taste and connoisseurship: visual reflex is stronger than intellectual reflection. (From Victor Vasarely: Victor Vasarely [Werner Spies, ed.]. New York, Harry N. Abrams, Inc., 1971.)

practitioner has the opportunity to treat a major occlusal disharmony early, treatment is less complicated and the results are usually more successful.

The practicing dentist must always keep in mind that there is an optimal time for the treatment of minor and major occlusal disharmonies. This can only be accomplished by careful examination of the occlusal relationships of the primary, mixed and permanent dentitions.

It is the aim of this text to provide factual, clear information, so that the dental practitioner may recognize and treat minor occlusal disharmonies early in the developing dentition. In this way the pediatric dentist and the general practitioner will carry out the true aims of prevention and provide the growing child with a satisfactory functional dentition.

M. MICHAEL COHEN, SR.

ACKNOWLEDGMENTS

Numerous young colleagues have made possible the preparation of this book by their untiring assistance.

I am particularly grateful to Drs. Bruce Fieldman, Richard M. Reiter and Gregory M. Shupik for their generous help. To Dr. Leonard J. Carapezza go special thanks for the loan of many casts of cases requiring treatment for minor occlusal disharmonies. To Drs. Don Occaso and Orlando Rodríguez-Rams I extend my appreciation, and to Drs. Eugene E. West and J. Rodney Mathews my gratitude for the loan of casts showing the results of early treatment of occlusal disharmonies.

A sincere acknowledgment is made to the following practitioners, who have reviewed parts of the text and made many valuable suggestions:

Dr. Joseph Keller, Associate Professor of Pedodontics, New York University, School of Dentistry.

Dr. David H. Watson, Milwaukee, Wisconsin.

My appreciation goes to the following photographers, art designers and dental laboratories for their contribution to the text:

Richard W. St. Clair, F.P.S.A., Brookline, Massachusetts.

Arrco Medical Art & Design, Inc., Brookline, Massachusetts.

The Cettel Studio, Inc., Chestertown, New York.

Study Models, Inc., Charles Daniels, C.D.T., Roxbury, Massachusetts.

Warren M. Sheridan, Laboratory Technician, Children's Hospital Medical Center, Boston, Massachusetts.

Space Maintainers Laboratory, Panorama City, California.

To Dr. Louise G. Cohen, my daughter-in-law, I give special thanks for her help in editing the text. I am particularly grateful to my Executive Secretary, Tilla Fishman, for typing the manuscript.

M.M.C., Sr.

SPECIAL ACKNOWLEDGMENT

I wish to thank the entire staff of the W. B. Saunders Company for their interest and enthusiasm in the preparation of this text. They were at all times available and were unusually helpful in the meticulous preparation of the illustrations and text.

M. MICHAEL COHEN, SR.

CONTENTS

6

RECOGNITION, DIAGNOSIS AND TREATMENT OF CLASS II OCCLUSAL DISHARMONIES

7

MINOR TOOTH MOVEMENT IN THE EARLY AND MIXED PERMANENT DENTITIONS

1

Practical Considerations

I have deliberately deleted the words "normal" and "ideal" from this text. When Angle propounded his classification of malocclusion he based it on several skulls in which ideal occlusion appeared to exist.

He stated in the introduction to his text, *Malocclusion of the Teeth,* that "no two normal human dentures have been created that were exactly alike; it is reasonable to suppose that since it has never yet been demonstrated that Nature ever duplicates her forms." Angle did not realize that the ideal rarely or never exists in nature, and yet the terms "normal" and "ideal" are profusely used in dental literature today. This concept of ideal occlusion has permeated the entire field of dentistry, not only in the area of orthodontics but also in the province of fixed and removable prostheses. When one examines large numbers of young children one rarely finds an ideal occlusion in the primary, mixed or permanent dentitions. What one finds is simply an occlusion that exists in a child, and it is with this concept in mind that this text is written, to better understand the child and the particular occlusal relationships that occur in childhood. Rather than use the terms "normal" or "ideal," I believe it is much more accurate to use the term "satisfactory," since the ideal is almost nonexistent in the dentition of a growing child.

I have also deleted from this text as much as possible the word "malocclusion," since it connotes a condition that may have pathological overtones. What is termed a malocclusion has no pathological manifestations either in the jaw bones or in the periodontium. In its place I have chosen to use "occlusal disharmonies," since this term describes occlusal relationships that are not in harmony with the developing dentition. An occlusal disharmony is a variation of occlusal relationships that frequently manifests itself as a dentofacial deformity not unlike a hooked nose or pitcher ears. Occlusal disharmonies therefore are treated primarily to improve the craniofacial and dentofacial relationships. The aim in treating minor occlusal disharmonies is to guide the teeth into their proper occlusal relationships using the child's natural occlusion as a means for achieving the maximum growth and development of the dentition.

1

FABRICATION OF APPLIANCES

In this text I do not intend to describe in detail the fabrication of a removable or fixed appliance but rather to give a descriptive illustration or drawing of it. Many practitioners prefer to fabricate their own appliances; this is their prerogative. In the References following most chapters and in the Suggested Readings at the end of the book are listed texts devoted to the fabrication of appliances. However, I believe that the time has come when the practitioner should utilize all of his time treating his patients and allow a competent certified laboratory technician to fabricate the appliances used for the treatment of a particular condition. Seamless bands

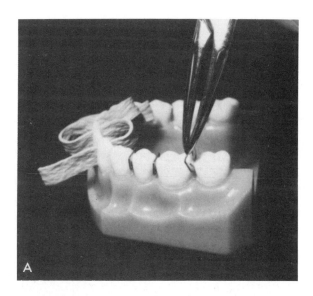

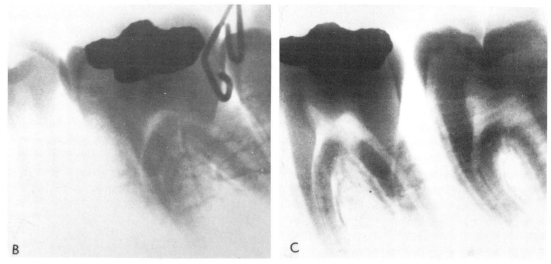

Figure 1–1

A, Separator placed between the teeth. The separators are inserted from the buccal side.
B, Roentgenogram showing separator in the embrasure.
C, Roentgenogram on day after separation.
(Courtesy of Dental Corporation of America, Washington, D.C.)

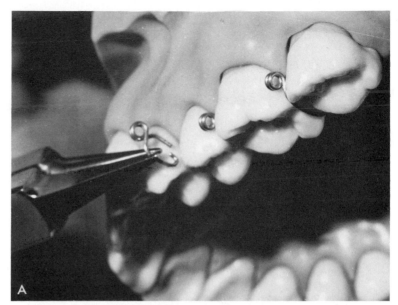

Figure 1–2

A, TP self-locking separating springs shown placed between the teeth.

B, Large size self-locking separating spring for use between molars. (A smaller size is used between premolars and canines.) (Courtesy of TP Laboratories, Inc., LaPorte, Indiana.)

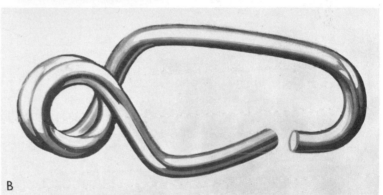

and stainless steel crowns are made accurately in standard sizes, so that it is not difficult for the dental practitioner to adapt them to teeth for appliance therapy. It is important that the practitioner be familiar with the materials necessary for fabricating an appliance. In addition, it is essential that he or she know how to write a prescription for the appliance so that the technician can understand how to make it.

The following procedure is recommended when removable appliances are to be fabricated by a dental laboratory:

1. Alginate impressions are satisfactory for removable appliances and it is suggested that they be poured immediately in stone.

2. New impressions should always be taken and a new model made for repairs and remakes.

3. A wax bite is very useful in establishing occlusal relationships. Impression in rubber base or silicone may be taken when indirect banding is desired. Stainless steel or precious metal bands may be used but require additional chair time.

Before direct or indirect bands are placed, the use of separating wire

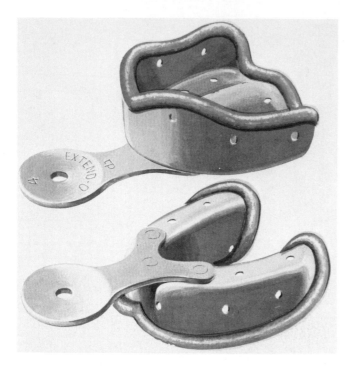

Figure 1–3. Maxillary and mandibular T.P. Teflon Extend-O-Trays. (Courtesy of TP Laboratories, Inc., LaPorte, Indiana.)

simplifies the placement of the band. D.C.A. separators are self-locking separating springs and are easily placed; these may stay between the teeth for several days or longer without causing severe gingival inflammation.

Figure 1–1 shows separating wires placed between the teeth, and Figure 1–2 illustrates T.P. self-locking separating springs. Extend-O-Trays, because of their design (Fig. 1–3), may be used effectively for taking impressions not only of the teeth but of the soft tissues as well. These trays are Teflon coated and allow for accurate impressions. Impression material is readily removed from the tray, leaving a smooth surface, and makes cleansing of the tray easy.

CLASPS (Fig. 1–4*A* to *F*)

Clasps depend on undercuts for resistance to displacement of removable appliances. The clasp material is made to fit below such undercuts and grasp the tooth. The undercuts that may be utilized for clasping surfaces may be found buccally, lingually, mesially and distally on primary molars, premolars and permanent molars, and mesially and distally on canines and incisors.

Figure 1–4 (*A* to *F*) illustrates the more common types of clasps used for removable appliances.

C Clasps (Fig. 1–4*A*)

Retention: Fair. This type usually is not recommended for primary retention but is a good auxiliary clasp. The tooth must be fully erupted so

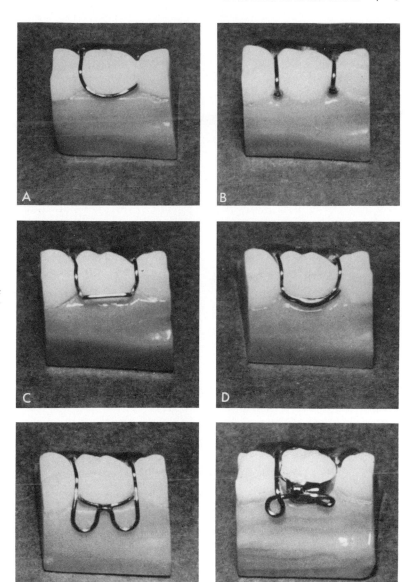

Figure 1–4. Illustrations of the more common types of clasps for retention of removable appliances (see text). (Courtesy of Space Maintainers Laboratory, Panorama City, California.)

that the clasp may seat under the mesial or distal surface of the buccal undercuts.

Ball Clasps (Fig. 1–4*B*)

Retention: Fair to good. Ball clasps fit into the interproximal area, usually between two teeth. This type lacks stability as a primary source of retention but makes an excellent auxiliary clasp. It is used between molars and premolars.

Adams Clasps (Modified Arrowhead) (Fig. 1–4C)

Retention: Best universal clasp. Adams clasps are both retentive and stable, easy to adjust, and neat and comfortable. They are used on bicuspids, premolars and erupted molars, and cause a minimum of bite disturbance.

Crozat Clasps (Fig. 1–4D)

Retention: Good to excellent. This type is a modification of the Jackson crib clasp, which uses the medial distal surface of buccal undercuts for retention. It is best suited for fully erupted molars when stability is essential.

Sage Clasps (Fig. 1–4E)

Retention: Good to excellent. Sage clasps use the medial distal surfaces of both buccal and lingual undercuts for retention. They are easy to adjust and very stable. These are excellent for partially erupted molars and premolars.

Band and Bar Clasps (Fig. 1–4F)

Retention: Excellent. These are banded to the molar or premolar and have buccal bar extensions from the retainers to hook on the band surface. They can be used on partially erupted teeth.

LABIAL ARCH WIRES (Fig. 1–5A to D)

There are many types of labial arch wires. Figure 1–5 illustrates the more common types that may be utilized for retention or for treatment when removable appliance therapy is indicated.

Round Arch Wire (Fig. 1–5A)

The most versatile type of labial arch (Hawley) wire, this type affords anterior retention, guidance for moving teeth and support for addition of attachments and finger springs. It can pass over occlusion at the distal surface of cuspids or first bicuspids.

Flat Contour Wire (Fig. 1–5B)

This arch wire consists of a section of flat wire contoured to the anterior surfaces from cuspid to cuspid. It is used in final retainers to

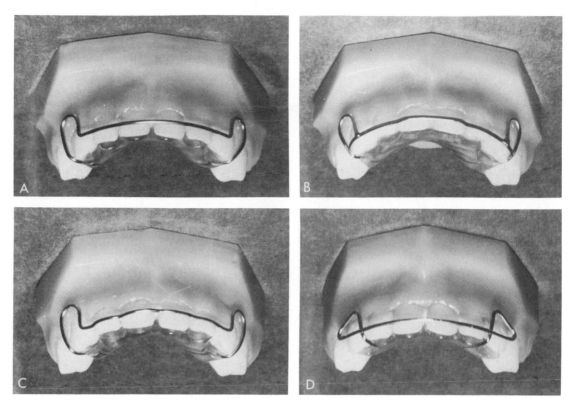

Figure 1–5. Labial arch wires (see text).

stabilize teeth when cuspid support is also desirable. It passes over the occlusion distal to the cuspids.

Round Contour Wire (Fig. 1–5*C*)

This type is the same as round labial wire but is contoured around specified teeth to prevent space closure while maintaining the same position. Usually it passes over the occlusion distal to the cuspids. It can be used on final retainers and is more retentive than regular round arch labials.

1 × 4 Round Wire (Fig. 1–5*D*)

This type is used as retaining wire when cuspids and bicuspids are being moved distally, precluding the use of a regular round labial arch wire. The wire passes between the cuspid and the lateral surface, going over the occlusion.

PRESCRIPTION BLANK

An example of a prescription blank for the technician to follow for fabricating appliances is shown in Figure 1–6.

PLEASE INDICATE ADDRESS CHANGES

☐ Send Mailing Materials

DATE WANTED

℞ Please Check Below:

UPPER	LOWER	APPLIANCE TYPE
☐	☐	Removable (Schwarz)
☐	☐	Fixed Band
☐	☐	Crozat: ☐ Gold ☐ Elgiloy
☐	☐	Temporary Partial
☐	☐	Functional – Check Below

FUNCTIONAL APPLIANCES

☐ Bimler-Type ____________
☐ Mono Block Activator
☐ Grind in above
☐ Modified Activator
☐ Oral Screen
☐ Frankel-Type ____________
☐ Bruxism Splint - Acrylic
☐ Bruxism Splint - Vacuum
☐ Athletic Mouthguard
☐ Positioner

PLEASE USE REVERSE SIDE FOR OTHER INSTRUCTIONS →

* Note: Work models are damaged beyond use in processing and cannot be returned. Please pour two sets or check "Duplicate Models" if you desire an extra set.

PATIENT'S FULL NAME (IMPORTANT–PLEASE PRINT) AGE

DOCTOR'S SIGNATURE ______________________ D.D.S.

License No. ______________ Today's Date ______________

℞ ✓PLEASE CHECK APPLIANCE TYPE ON REVERSE SIDE

NOTE—WORK MODELS CANNOT BE RETURNED—SEE OTHER SIDE

DESIGN CASE HERE

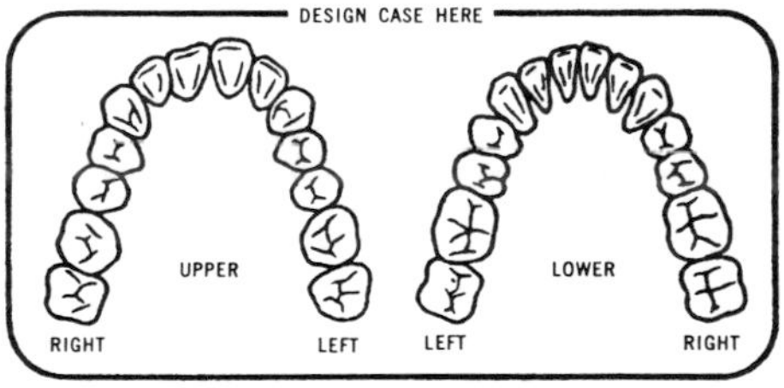

Figure 1–6. A sample prescription blank. *Left,* front part of prescription; *right,* back of prescription.

CORRECTION OF BILATERAL CROSSBITE

A removable appliance is used for the correction of a bilateral posterior crossbite involving the maxillary right and left first and second primary molars (Fig. 1–7*A*).

Prescription. Maxillary Schwartz expansion appliance with Adams clasps on maxillary second molar. Ball clasps between first primary molar and primary canines, labial arch wire from canine to canine (Fig. 1–7*B*).

CORRECTION OF POSTERIOR CROSSBITE

Bands for correction of unilateral or bilateral posterior crossbite of primary or permanent dentition are prescribed (Fig. 1–8*A*).

Prescription. Band the maxillary and mandibular right first permanent molars with hooks or buttons for attaching cross elastics to correct crossbite (Fig. 1–8*B*).

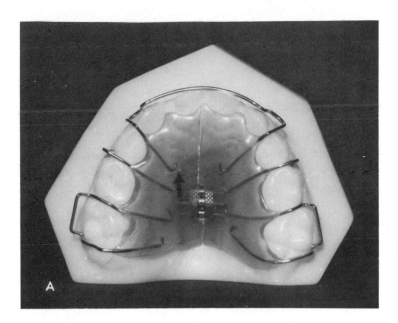

Figure 1–7. Correction of bilateral crossbite (see text).

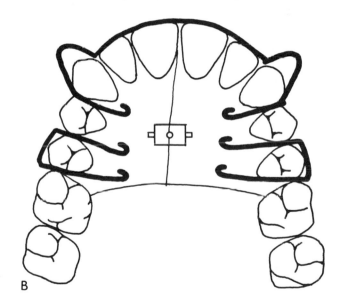

FIXED MAXILLARY EXPANSION APPLIANCE

Fixed maxillary expansion appliance is used to correct posterior crossbite involving molars or molars and canines (Fig. 1–9*A*).

Prescription. Bands on primary canines and primary second molars. Acrylic palate and expansion screw (Fig. 1–9*B*). This appliance is cemented on teeth and remains in place for several months after expansion has been accomplished to prevent relapse of crossbite.

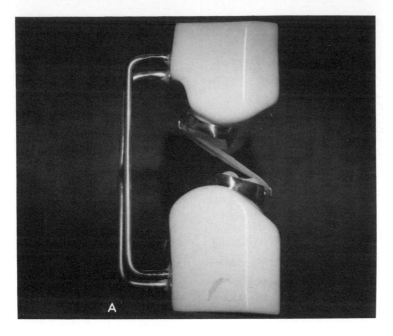

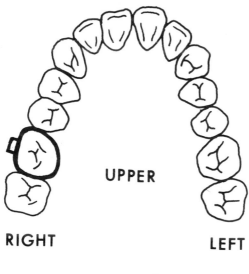

UPPER

RIGHT   LEFT

LOWER

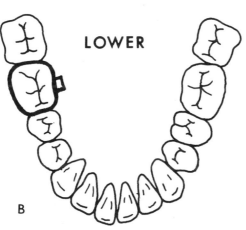

Figure 1–8. Correction of posterior crossbite (see text).

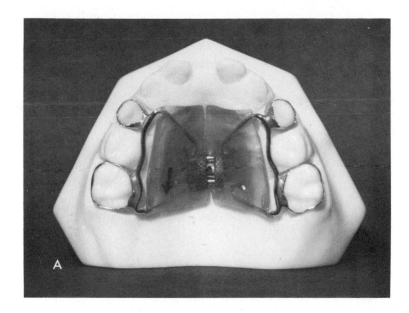

Figure 1–9. Fixed maxillary expansion appliance (see text).

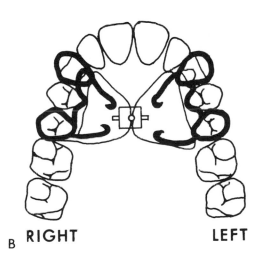

B RIGHT   LEFT

INSTRUCTIONS FOR WEARING ELASTICS*

The following are suggestions for patients who wear elastics for tooth movement and orthodontic treatment.

1. The size of the elastics is written on the package of envelopes. Remember the size you wear and if you find yourself without elastics between appointments write or come to the office for a fresh supply.

2. Wear the elastics all the time except when you eat or brush your

---

*As suggested by Dr. William H. Williams, Athens, Georgia.

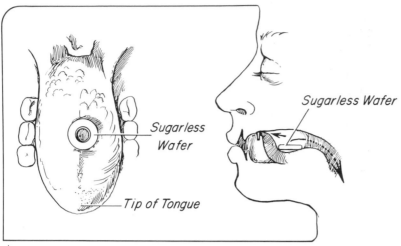

A

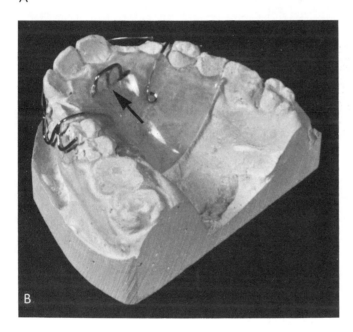

B

Figure 1–10. Sugarless wafer exercise for controlling tongue thrust and other tongue deviations (see text).

teeth. Do not eat anything with elastics in your mouth, because this causes the appliance to loosen or break. Gum chewing with elastics will also loosen or break the appliance.

3. The elastics should be changed four times a day; a fresh pair should be inserted in the morning after breakfast, after lunch, after dinner, and before retiring at night.

The dentist will give you instructions on the number of elastics to be worn; in most instances one elastic is worn on each side of the mouth. If a band becomes loose or the appliance breaks, elastics should not be worn until the appliance is repaired.

When elastics are first worn the teeth may be tender and painful. This soreness may last several days, after which it will disappear.

The greatest and best results for the correction of occlusal dishar-monies are obtained by wearing the elastics at all times, day and night, and changing the elastics *four times a day.*

SUGARLESS WAFER EXERCISE FOR CONTROLLING TONGUE THRUST AND OTHER TONGUE DEVIATIONS*

1. Place sugarless wafer on back of tongue (Fig. 1–10*A*).
2. Lift tongue until sugarless wafer touches roof of your mouth.
3. Place the tip of the tongue behind the bar indicated by the arrow on the removable acrylic habit reminder (Fig. 1–10*B*).
4. As the sugarless wafer melts, swallow, but do not allow your tongue to move from behind the bar.
5. Continue the exercise until the entire sugarless wafer has melted.
6. Do this exercise at least three times a day.
7. Keep a chart, such as the following:

Date	Times
June 1	(Record the number of times you did the exercise)
June 2	
June 3	

8. Bring the chart and package of sugarless wafers to all appointments.
9. When swallowing always place the tip of your tongue behind the tongue guard.
10. Do not perform this exercise in the presence of other people or while watching television.
11. Do not do this exercise sitting up or lying down. Perform it in a reclining (half sitting) position.

---

*From the instructions form of Dr. William A. Williams, Athens, Georgia.

2
Radiography for Pediatric Dentistry

It is essential to have a complete radiographic survey for a thorough diagnosis in pediatric dentistry. There are certain considerations that should determine the number of radiographs necessary to view all areas of the dentofacial complex that are involved in a diagnosis.

SURVEYS FOR PRESCHOOL CHILDREN (AGES 2 TO 5 YEARS)

A radiographic survey for a preschool child utilizes No. 0 film, which is small enough to place in a young child's mouth (Fig. 2–1). The survey

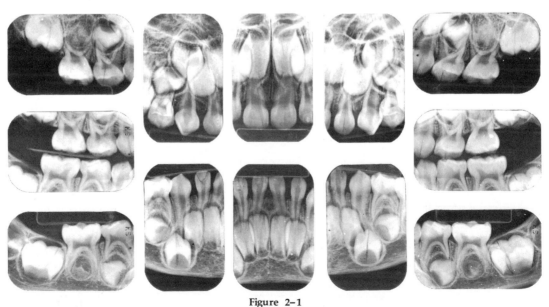

Figure 2–1

(From Silha, R. E.: Dental Radiography and Photography, Vol. 45, No. 2, 1972. Courtesy of Eastman Kodak Company.)

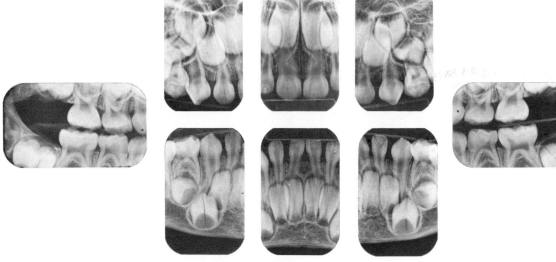

Figure 2-2
(Courtesy of Eastman Kodak Company.)

includes three films for the mandibular anterior region, three films for the maxillary anterior area, one film for the right molar and one film for the left molar areas. Two posterior bite-wing films, one for the right side and the other for the left side, complete the survey.

Another type of survey utilizes No. 0 film in the anterior areas of the maxilla and mandible (Fig. 2-2). For the posterior area, two No. 1 films are utilized, one for the right molar area and the second for the left molar area.

In Figure 2-3, No. 0 film is used for the anterior maxillary and mandibular areas, and an occlusal film is utilized for an extraoral posterior lateral jaw view. This type of survey may be used for very young patients when they cannot tolerate the placement of film in the posterior areas.

Figure 2-4 illustrates a survey by Silha (1972) that covers extensive areas of the mouth and yet requires relatively little cooperation from the patient. The survey utilizes three occlusal films folded in the middle with a lead barrier between the two film surfaces. This technique consists of taking occlusal projections for the maxillary and mandibular anterior and posterior areas. By folding the film and using a lead barrier, the film need be positioned for only three areas—the anterior and the right and left posterior areas. Once the film has been positioned for each area, two exposures may be made without removing the film from the mouth. A 1/16 in. thick wafer of lead will prevent the radiation from penetrating and fogging the film to be used for the opposite arch.

The very young child usually can accommodate film placement better if he has something to bite upon, such as the film or a film-positioning device. The amount of radiographic coverage needed may be determined by the cooperation of the very young patient.

Figure 2-5 shows the use of four No. 2 films for a survey that is very easy to make for the very young child. This survey was suggested by Waggener and Ireland (1953). The No. 2 film is used for the occlusal

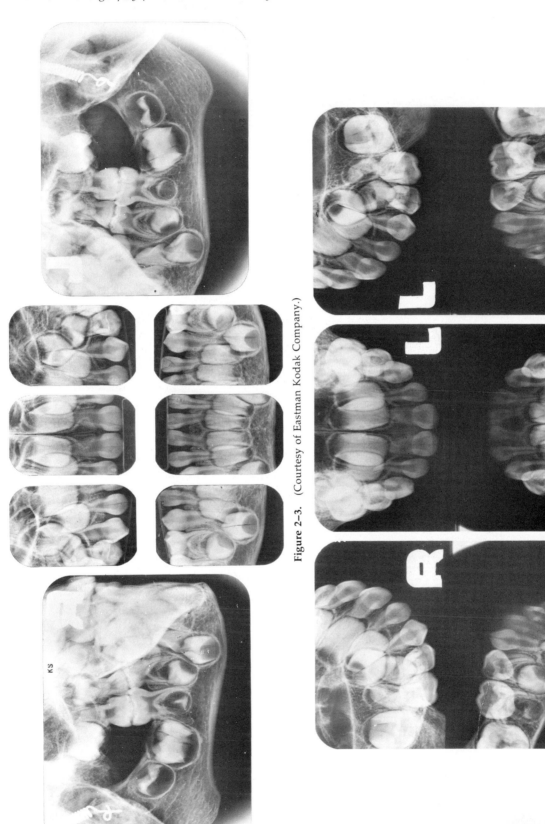

Figure 2–3. (Courtesy of Eastman Kodak Company.)

Figure 2–4. (Courtesy of Eastman Kodak Company.)

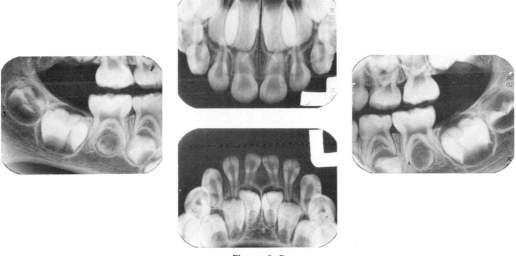

Figure 2–5

(Courtesy of Eastman Kodak Company.)

projections of the anterior areas in the maxilla and mandible. Then No. 0, No. 1 or No. 2 film can be used for the posterior bite-wing examination, depending on the size of the dental arch, the age of the patient and the degree of patient cooperation. This simple survey yields quite a bit of information for having used only four radiographs. As a preliminary screening survey or as an introduction for the young patient, it is very useful.

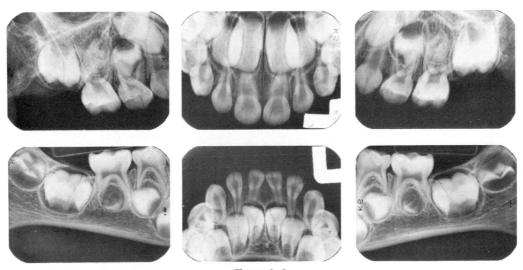

Figure 2–6

(Courtesy of Eastman Kodak Company.)

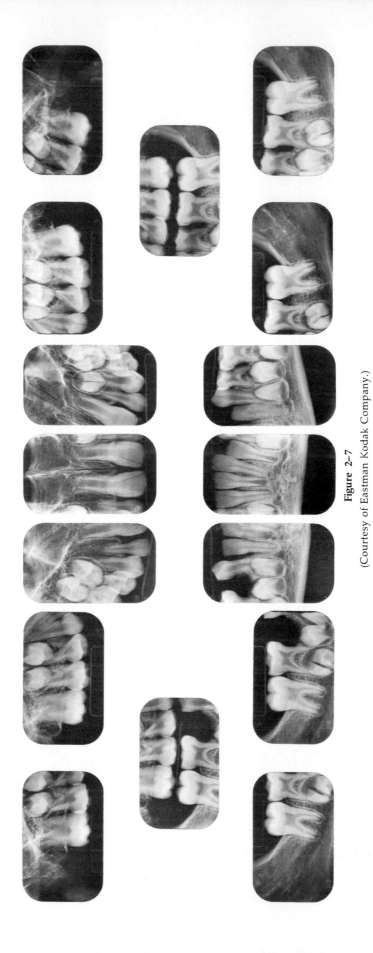

Figure 2-7

(Courtesy of Eastman Kodak Company.)

SURVEYS FOR CHILDREN OF AGES 6 TO 12 YEARS IN PEDIATRIC DENTISTRY

As the child grows older, he can understand and cooperate to a greater extent, and usually the size of the mouth enlarges, which allows the use of larger x-ray film. Figure 2–7 illustrates a very useful intermediate radiographic survey for this age group. The entire survey is made with No. 1 film, which yields sufficient information for children of this size and yet does facilitate film placement because it is smaller than the No. 2 film. Most of the children in this age group accommodate placement of the films very well. A variation might be the use of No. 2 film instead of the No. 1 for the posterior bite-wing examinations. This arrangement of 14 films, which does not include the posterior bite-wing films and which uses No. 2 film for all areas, was recommended by Morgan and undoubtedly by many others. However, the placement of films for the anterior areas is greatly facilitated by using the No. 1 film.

The children in this age group have mixed dentitions, and a larger size of film than the No. 0 should be used as soon as possible. In the older children, two posterior bite-wing films for each side may be required.

Figure 2–8 illustrates the survey that can be used for the older children in this age group. The No. 2 film does yield greater coverage in the posterior areas of the mouth and may result in greater diagnostic yield. It is important to be able to see as much of the developing permanent teeth as possible. The children with mixed dentitions need careful

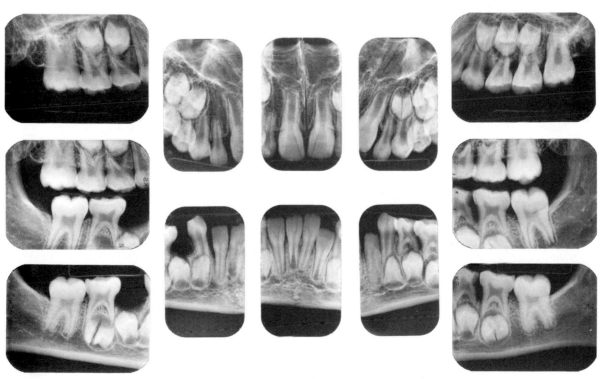

Figure 2–8
(Courtesy of Eastman Kodak Company.)

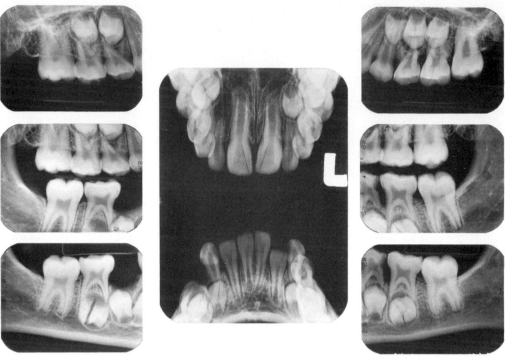

Figure 2–9

(Courtesy of Eastman Kodak Company.)

examination in order to diagnose developmental aberrations of the permanent dentition as soon as possible. The coverage in this survey is adequate.

Figure 2–9 shows an interesting variation of a survey that could be made for the 6 to 12 year age group. The occlusal film can be folded, and two radiographs can be made from one film. When these radiographs are used in combination with the No. 2 radiographs of the molar and posterior areas, they provide a very informative survey. Many times it is surprising how much information can be gained from a comparatively small number of films when it is necessary to compromise because of some of the factors previously mentioned. Although the anterior areas are not quite as well covered as in Figures 2–7 and 2–8, they probably would be adequate for an initial screening survey.

Figure 2–10 shows an interesting survey that can be obtained with very few films. No. 2 films are used for the anterior incisor areas, and occlusal films are used for the posterior lateral jaw projections. If the size of the patient's mouth is fairly small, No. 1 films could be substituted for No. 2 films. The redeeming feature of this survey is the small amount of patient cooperation required. Even with an uncooperative child, it should be possible to make the two anterior periapical radiographs.

Figure 2–11 shows the use of occlusal radiographs for all the areas of the mouth. As was shown in Figure 2–4 with the smaller patient, this survey could be used if it were found necessary to compromise to the point that this was the only intraoral radiographic evaluation that could be obtained.

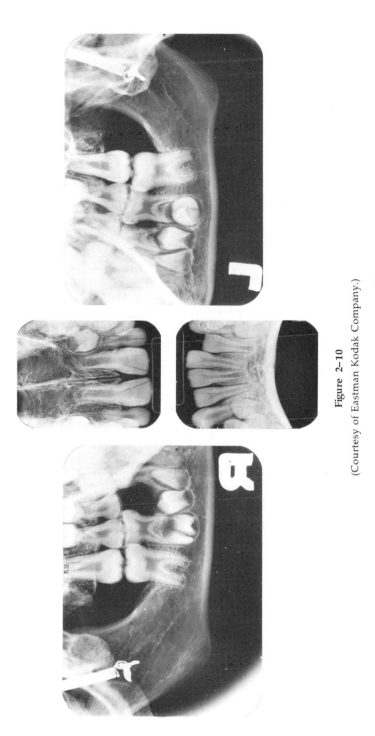

Figure 2–10
(Courtesy of Eastman Kodak Company.)

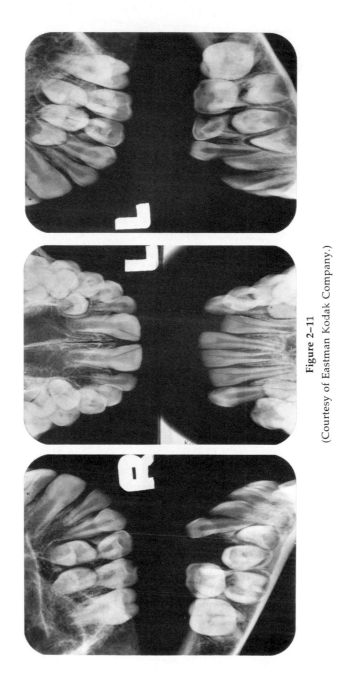

Figure 2–11
(Courtesy of Eastman Kodak Company.)

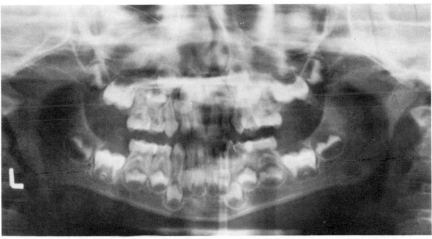

Figure 2–12. Panoramic radiograph from a boy 4 years of age. Note that 28 permanent teeth are present. (Courtesy of Robert E. Silha and Eastman Kodak Company.)

PANORAMIC RADIOGRAPHY

Panoramic radiography complements intraoral roentgenography and is not intended to replace the complete intraoral roentgenographic survey. The advantage of panoramic radiography is the comprehensive scope of the visualization of the teeth, their supporting structures, the entire maxilla and mandible and the adjacent structures. Projection of the teeth in their correct relationship to adjacent anatomic structures and to each other is invaluable in pediatric dentistry, orthodontics and oral surgery.

Figures 2–12 through 2–17 are panoramic radiographs of children showing the primary, mixed and permanent dentitions.

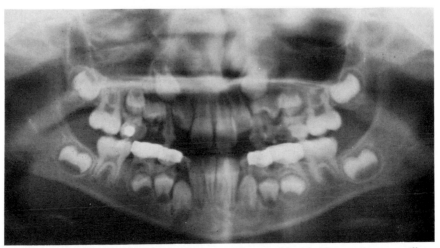

Figure 2–13. Panoramic radiograph from a 7 year old girl. Note carious maxillary primary molars and stainless steel crowns on mandibular molars. (Courtesy of Robert E. Silha and Eastman Kodak Company.)

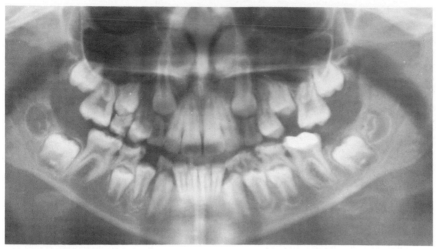

Figure 2–14. Panoramic radiograph from a 9 year old girl. Note carious primary molars in maxilla and mandible.

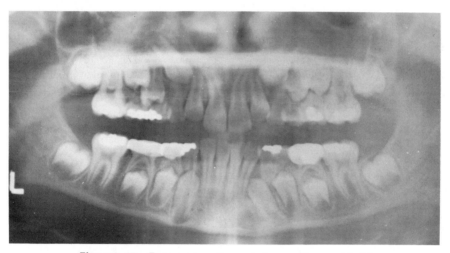

Figure 2–15. Panoramic radiograph from a 10 year old girl.

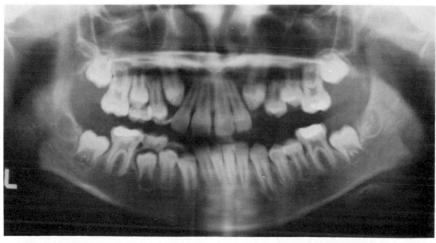

Figure 2–16. Panoramic radiograph from an 11 year old girl. Note carious primary molars with space loss in maxillary and mandibular premolar areas.

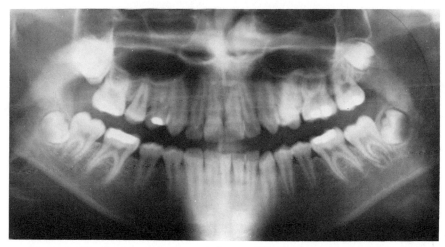

Figure 2–17. Panoramic radiograph from a 13½ year old boy. Note good alignment of dentition and the presence of maxillary and mandibular third molars.

REFERENCES

Bachman, L. H.: Pedodontic radiography. Dental Radiography and Photography. Vol. 44, Number 3. Rochester, N.Y., Eastman Kodak Company, 1971.

Berkman, M. D.: Pedodontic radiographic interpretation. Dental Radiography and Photography. Vol. 44, Number 2. Rochester, N.Y., Eastman Kodak Company, 1971.

Christen, A. G., and Segreto, V. A.: Distortion and artifacts encountered in Panorex radiography. J.A.D.A., 77:1096–1101, 1968.

Cohen, M. M.: Pediatric Dentistry. 2nd Ed. St. Louis, C. V. Mosby Co., 1961.

Doykos, J. D., III: Pedodontic radiography. *In* Current Dental Therapy. St. Louis, C. V. Mosby Co., 1974.

Doykos, J. D., III: The necessity for full mouth radiographs in dentistry for children. J. Mass. Dental Soc., 18:85–89, 1969.

Graber, T. M.: Panoramic radiography in dentistry. J. Canad. Dent. Assoc., 31:158, 1965.

Graber, T. M.: Panoramic radiography in orthodontic diagnosis. Am. J. Orthod., 53:799–821, 1967.

Law, D. B., et al.: An Atlas of Pedodontics. Philadelphia, W. B. Saunders Company, 1969.

Silha, R. E.: Special radiographic surveys. Dental Radiography and Photography. Vol. 45, Number 2. Rochester, N.Y., Eastman Kodak Company, 1972.

Updegrave, W. J.: Panoramic dental radiograph. Dental Radiography and Photography. Vol. 36, Number 4. Rochester, N.Y., Eastman Kodak Company, 1963.

Updegrave, W. J.: The role of panoramic radiography in diagnosis. Oral Surg., 22:49, 1966.

Waggener, D. T., and Ireland, R. L.: Intraoral roentgenography for children. J.A.D.A., 47:133–139, 1953.

3

Cephalometric Roentgenography in Pediatric Dentistry

GERALD BORELL

It is difficult to determine the severity of an occlusal disharmony without the information available from a roentgenographic cephalogram. The cephalogram enables the dentist to more accurately determine craniofacial and dentofacial relationships. Cephalometric roentgenograms and dental casts are essential for the identification of severe occlusal disharmonies. The cephalometric roentgenograms make it possible to distinguish more precisely between a major and minor occlusal disharmony. The practitioner may then proceed to treat minor occlusal disharmonies for the prevention of major occlusal disharmonies.

Cephalograms are precisely oriented lateral or posterior-anterior radiographic plates. The lateral cephalogram is used much more frequently than the posterior-anterior cephalogram. Cephalograms are obtained by positioning the patient's head so that the median sagittal plane of the head is parallel to the plane of the film and perpendicular to the central ray of the radiation emanating from the x-ray tube.

The head is oriented by adjustable rods that fit snugly into the external auditory meatuses. The lowest point on the rim of the left orbit is palpated and the head is rotated around the ear rod axis until this point is at the same level as the top of the ear rods.

Since x-ray radiation diverges from the anode of the tube, the farther the anode is positioned away from the head the less divergent the rays will be and the less the image recorded on the film will be enlarged. The distance of 60 in. from the anode to the median sagittal plane of the patient's head is now standard. This distance reduces magnification to an acceptable range and keeps the dimensions of the cephalometer practical. Magnification is also affected by the distance from the head to the plane of the film. Thus, the film is placed close to the head, usually at a fixed distance (Fig. 3–1).

26

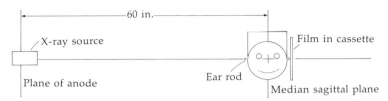

Figure 3–1. The cephalometer is composed of a cephalostat, or head stabilizer, and a device to precisely align and hold the x-ray source. The cephalostat orients and stabilizes the head so that an axis passing through the patient's ears is aligned with the central ray of radiation. The lowest point of the left orbit is brought by the dentist into the same horizontal plane as the top of the ear rods. A standard 90 KV (kilovolts) dental x-ray machine is an adequate source of radiation. At 90 KV and 15 m.a. (milliamperes) an exposure time of 0.5 sec. is usually appropriate. Proper collimation is important so that only the radiation needed to expose the film passes through the patient and all other radiation is blocked.

Since the x-ray tube is positioned at a considerable distance from the patient, the exposure time required to obtain a satisfactory image becomes significant. Involuntary movement by the patient over this time would blur the image on the film. To reduce the time, the film is exposed in a cassette in which the film is sandwiched between two intensifying screens. These screens emit light when exposed to x-ray radiation. The film is thus exposed both by the radiation passing through it and by the light from the screens that are exposed to the same radiation. Most of the exposure of the film is caused by the light emitted by the screens (Fig. 3–2). The processed film shows images of the hard tissue and structures of the head and neck, as well as numerous soft tissue structures, and provides a soft tissue profile.

After careful examination of the film to observe the relationship of hard and soft tissues, a tracing is made. A thin translucent plastic sheet

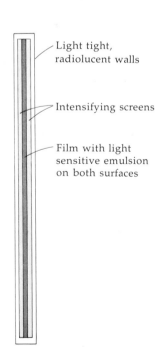

Figure 3–2. Cross section of a film cassette. The exposure time of the film is significantly reduced by employing a cassette with intensifying screens. The cassette is a light tight box that can accommodate a sheet of 8 × 10 in. x-ray film. Kodak Blue Brand or an equivalent film is used. This film is sensitive to exposure to both x-ray radiation and light. The radiation that passes through the patient's head when making a cephalogram takes the following course: It penetrates the radiolucent front wall of the cassette, the front intensifying screen, the film and the back intensifying screen, and exits through the rear wall of the cassette. The intensifying screens fluoresce when exposed to radiation and emit light. The amount of light emitted by the intensifying screens at a given point is proportional to the intensity of x-ray radiation at that point. Any paper covering the film must be removed to permit the film to be exposed to the light emitted by the screens. The exposure of the film is achieved primarily by the light emitted by the screens and secondarily by the x-ray radiation acting directly on the film.

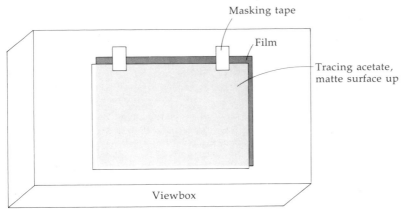

Figure 3–3. Preparing to trace the cephalogram. A thin plastic sheet with a matte finish on one surface is taped down to the film and to the viewbox with the matte surface up. Masking tape is satisfactory. The tape is placed only on the superior edge of the plastic sheet, so that one could lift up the sheet to examine the film in order to identify more obscure regions. The film should project about ¼ in. beyond the plastic sheet so that the tape will hold the film also. Sometimes it is useful to block the light emitted by the viewbox beyond the edge of the film.

with a matte finish on one surface is taped down to the film and to the viewbox with the matte surface up. The outlines of the skeletal structures are then traced on the sheet with a sharp No. 2H pencil (Fig. 3–3).

The significant structures traced on the lateral cephalograms that may be used to evaluate the craniofacial and dentofacial relationships are as follows:

1. The soft tissue profile from the forehead to the outline of the chin.

2. The most anterior outline of the frontal bone and the outline of the nasal bones.

3. The outline of the maxilla—its anterior, nasal and oral surfaces—including the most prominent maxillary central incisor and the first permanent molar.

4. The outline of the mandible, the most prominent mandibular central incisor and the first permanent molar.

5. The outline of the rim of the orbit.

6. The outline of the ear rods.

7. The outline of sella turcica.

In tracing, the pencil is drawn on the outer outline of the bony structures where white lines or areas become black. The line is drawn so as to average all bilateral structures (Fig. 3–4).

The following hard tissue landmarks should be identified and marked on the tracings by dots or short lines perpendicular to the traced outline.

1. *Nasion* (N): The most anterior point on the suture between the nasal and frontal bones.

2. *Sella* (S): The center of area of sella turcica as determined by inspection.

3. *Porion* (machine registration): The highest point on the outline of the ear rods, corresponding to the highest points in the external auditory meatuses.

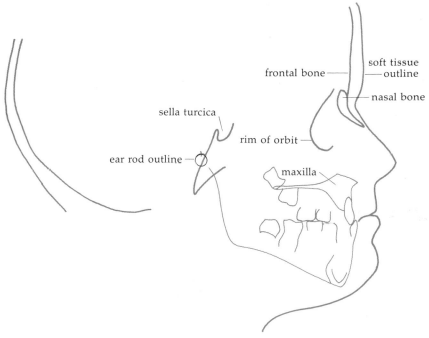

Figure 3–4. Structures of significance to be traced from the lateral cephalogram.

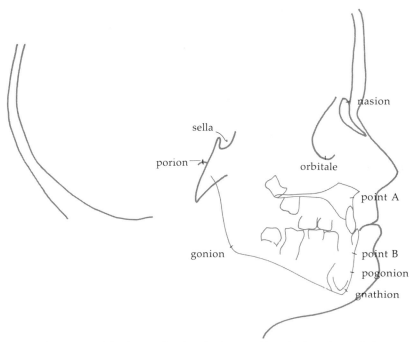

Figure 3–5. Hard tissue landmarks that are identified on the cephalogram and marked on the tracing.

4. *Orbitale*: The lowest point on the orbital margin.

5. *Point A*: The innermost point on the convexity of the anterior outline of the maxilla below the anterior nasal spine, usually at the level of the apices of the incisors.

6. *Point B*: The innermost point on the convexity of the anterior outline of the mandible, usually at the level of the apices of the incisors.

7. *Pogonion* (P): The most anterior point on the outline of the mandibular symphysis.

8. *Gnathion* (Gn): The outermost everted point on the mandibular symphysis.

9. *Gonion* (Go): The outermost everted point at the gonial angle of the mandible (Fig. 3–5).

Although there are many acceptable approaches to a quantitative analysis of the cephalogram, a modification of the Downs' Analysis is uncomplicated and useful in assessing an occlusal disharmony. Table 3–1 provides an example of mean values in a modified Downs' Analysis.

TABLE 3–1

	Children Mean S.D.
1. NP–Frankfort	89.4 ± 3.4
2. NAP	4.2 ± 5.4
3. SN–GoGn	32.3 ± 4.7
4. SGn–Frankfort	57.2 ± 3.3
5. SNA	80.8 ± 3.9
6. SNB	78.0 ± 3.1
7. Diff.	2.8
8. $\underline{1}$ to $\overline{1}$	130.4 ± 7.3
9. $\overline{1}$ to GoGn	93.5 ± 5.8
10. $\underline{1}$ to SN	103.5 ± 5.0

NP–Frankfort

The line from nasion to pogonion is termed the *facial plane*. The line from porion to orbitale is called the *Frankfort horizontal*. The intersection of these lines forms the *facial angle*. A large facial angle indicates a protrusion of the bony chin; conversely, a small angle indicates a retrusion of the chin (Fig. 3–6).

NAP

The angle formed by a line drawn from nasion to point A intersecting a line from point A to pogonion is called the *angle of convexity*. A flat

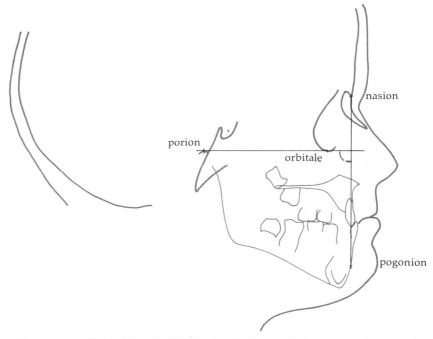

Figure 3–6. The facial angle (NP–Frankfort). (Figures 3–6 through 3–14 are of the first child described in the text, a 6 year old Caucasian girl.)

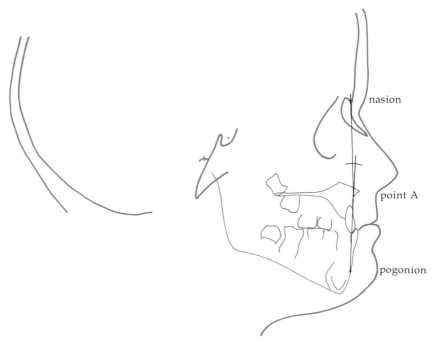

Figure 3–7. The angle of convexity (NAP).

profile means that the upper face (represented by nasion), the midface (represented by point A), and the chin (the pogonion) are on the same plane. A convex profile is caused by a protrusion of the maxilla or a retrusion of the mandible or both (or lack of a bony chin). A concave profile is caused by a retrusion of the maxilla or a protrusion of the mandible or both (Fig. 3–7).

SN–GoGn

The mandibular plane angle is formed by the line from gonion to gnathion, the mandibular plane, intersecting a line from sella to nasion. The line from sella to nasion represents the cranial base, a relatively stable area since growth in this region is completed early in life. A flat mandibular plane with a small mandibular angle is associated with a deep overbite. A steep mandibular plane and a large angle is correlated with a shallow overbite and, at the extreme, an open bite (Fig. 3–8).

SGn–Frankfort

A line from sella to gnathion is termed the Y axis. The angle formed as this line crosses the Frankfort horizontal plane can give the dentist an appreciation of the direction of growth of the lower face. A steep Y axis is indicative of a downward growing face, while a flatter axis is associated with a more forward growing face (Fig. 3–9).

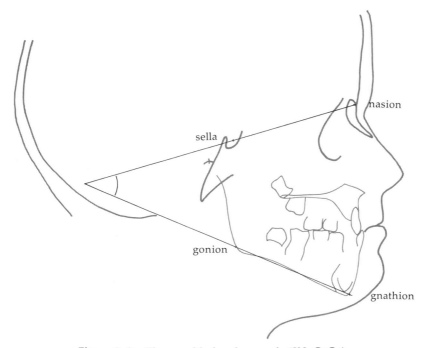

Figure 3–8. The mandibular plane angle (SN–GoGn).

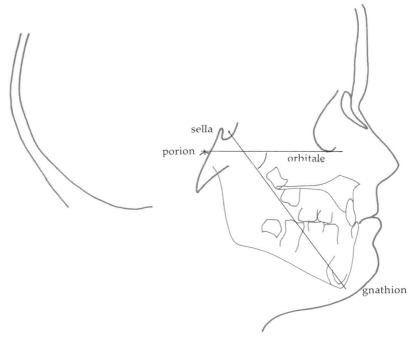

Figure 3–9. The angle formed by the Y axis and the Frankfort horizontal plane (SGn–FH).

SNA

The size of the angle formed by lines connecting the three points (sella, nasion and point A) is an indication of the relative protrusion or retrusion of the maxillary apical base (which is that bone that surrounds the apices of the maxillary teeth). The size of this angle should be correlated with the evaluation of size of the angle of convexity (Fig. 3–10).

SNB

The angle formed by connecting these points is an indication of protrusion or retrusion of the mandibular apical base. The evaluation of the magnitude of this angle should be done in conjunction with the evaluation of the facial angle and the angle of convexity (Fig. 3–11).

Diff.

The numerical difference between SNA and SNB is of considerable significance since it indicates the relative anteroposterior relationship of the bone supporting the maxillary teeth to the bone supporting the mandibular teeth. When this value is different from that given in Table 3–1 it indicates that difficulty might be expected in obtaining a good relationship of the maxillary incisors to the mandibular incisors.

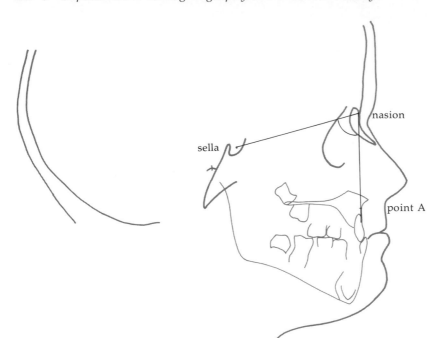

Figure 3–10. The anteroposterior relationship of the maxillary apical base (SNA).

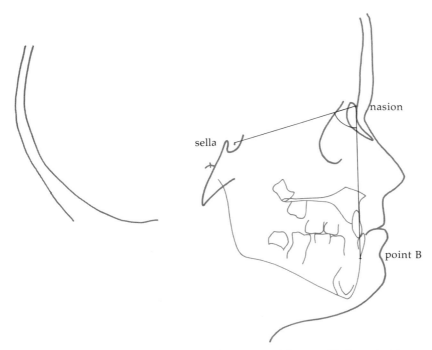

Figure 3–11. The anteroposterior relationship of the mandibular apical base (SNB).

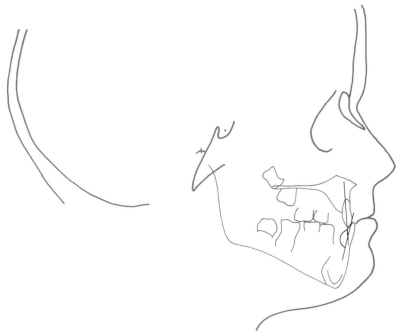

Figure 3–12. The angular relationship of the maxillary central incisors to the mandibular central incisors (1 to 1̄).

1 to 1̄

The angular relationship between the long axes of the most prominent maxillary and mandibular central incisors is of value only after evaluation of the relationship of these teeth to other planes (Fig. 3–12).

1̄ to GoGn

The size of the angle formed by the long axis of the mandibular central incisor and the mandibular plane indicates the extent to which these incisors are tipped labially or lingually. As the mandibular plane becomes steeper, it follows that the angular value should decrease to remain acceptable. The converse is also to be expected. A child whose mandibular plane is steep (37 degrees to Frankfort horizontal) would tend to have a 1̄ to GoGn angle of less than 90 degrees. Another child whose mandibular plane is shallow (28 degrees) might have a 1̄ to GoGn angle of 96 degrees. For each child the mandibular incisal angle that exists is acceptable (Fig. 3–13).

1 to SN

The axis of the most prominent maxillary central incisor and the sella-nasion line form an angle that indicates the extent of the labial or lingual inclination of these incisors (Fig. 3–14).

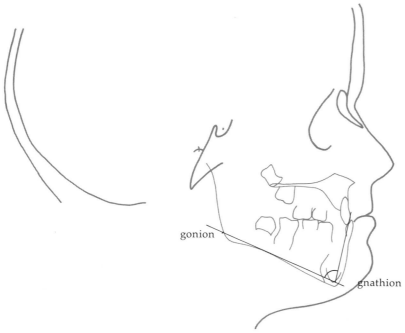

Figure 3–13. The angular relationship of the mandibular incisors to the mandibular plane (1̄ to GoGn).

When the angular values of the last three (1 to 1, 1̄ to GoGn, 1 to SN) vary significantly from the mean and the values for the first seven do not, the occlusal disharmony may be called a dental occlusal disharmony (with certain exceptions). When the values of some (or many) of the first seven vary significantly from the mean values, and an occlusal disharmony is present and is related to these variations from the mean, the occlusion can be termed a skeletal occlusal disharmony. Not all occlusal disharmonies can be evaluated and classified into dental or skeletal by an analysis that uses only a lateral cephalogram. Most skeletal occlusal disharmonies appear to involve variations from the normal, either anteroposteriorly or vertically. These are the dimensions displayed on the lateral cephalogram.

All measurements taken in this analysis are of angles. Angular relationships are not affected by the magnification present in every cephalogram, nor are they appreciably affected by distortion. Images of structures of the head that are not lying in planes perpendicular to the x-ray beam are always foreshortened; this foreshortening is termed distortion.

The following are examples of cephalometric analyses in young children:

Patient C.V. is a Caucasian girl aged 6 years 2 months (see Figures 3–6 to 3–14). Her primary dentition is complete. She has a lingual crossbite of all her maxillary anterior teeth and the left first and second primary molars. The midline of the maxillary and mandibular incisors is aligned on closure. There does not appear to be any sliding of the mandible forward to achieve maximal occlusal contact.

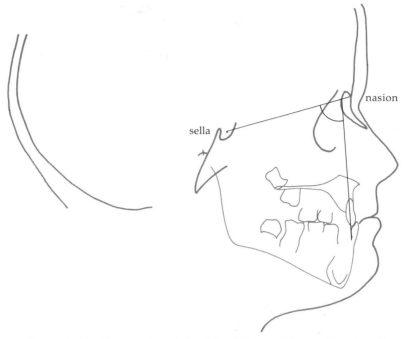

Figure 3–14. The angular relationship of the maxillary incisors to a line representing the anterior cranial base (1 to SN).

Note that the soft tissue profile shows an unesthetic relationship of the lower lip to the upper lip and a flattening of the soft tissue over the chin. The anterior crossbite and the tendency toward an Angle Class III relationship of the second primary molars may be observed.

Table 3–2 provides an analysis of the tracing.

Interpretation of this analysis indicates that the bony chin is in a satisfactory relationship anteroposteriorly since the facial angle is near the

TABLE 3–2

		Children Mean S.D.
NP–Frankfort	90	89.4 ± 3.4
NAP	4	4.2 ± 5.4
SN–GoGn	39	32.3 ± 4.7
SGn–Frankfort	53	57.2 ± 3.3
SNA	76	80.8 + 3.9
SNB	75	78.0 ± 3.1
Diff.	1	2.8
1 to 1	163	130.4 ± 7.3
1 to GoGn	78	93.5 ± 5.8
1 to SN	79	103.5 ± 5.0

mean. The face is relatively straight (slightly convex) since the angle of convexity is close to the mean.

The slope of the mandibular plane is somewhat steep, indicating a tendency toward an open bite pattern. The low value for the slope of the Y axis indicates a tendency for the mandible to grow forward more than usual.

It appears that sella turcica may be positioned more inferiorly than usual, since the angular values for SNA and SNB are both low. The anteroposterior position of the maxillary apical base may be considered to be relatively normal since the angle of convexity is close to the mean. Since the difference between SNA and SNB is small, the assumption would be that the mandibular apical base is located too far anteriorly.

A general summation of the analysis dealing with skeletal structures is that this child has a tendency toward mandibular prognathism.

The section of the analysis that deals with the dentition further supports this impression. The mandibular incisors are positioned too labially but are inclined lingually. The angular inclination of the maxillary incisor to the SN line as revealed by the analysis must be interpreted cautiously, since we have already established that this line may be slanted abnormally.

The second cephalometric analysis is of a Caucasian boy aged 7 years, 5 months (Figs. 3–15 and 3–16). He has an early mixed dentition. His first permanent molars are in occlusion. The occlusion on the right side is satisfactory and on the left side exhibits a Class II relationship. Several permanent incisors are erupting. There appears to be insufficient space for all of the permanent maxillary and mandibular incisors in the existing arches.

The soft tissue profile exhibits a deep sulcus below the lower lip. This is characteristic of insufficient facial height of the lower face. The side with the Class II molar relationship has been traced.

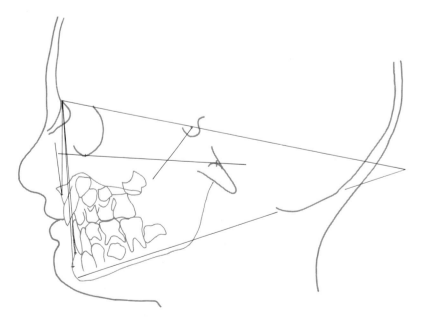

Figure 3–15. Angles used in the skeletal analysis of the second child described in the text, a 7 year old Caucasian boy.

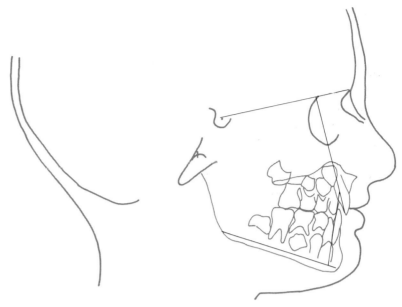

Figure 3–16. Angles used in the dental analysis of the 7 year old Caucasian boy described in the text.

The values obtained from an analysis of the tracing are as shown in Table 3–3.

The angular relationship of the facial plane to Frankfort horizontal indicates that the bony chin is retruded, implying a small bony chin or retrusion of the mandible. The angle of convexity is high—is the maxillary apical base too forward and the mandible retruded? Tentatively, based on the facial angle, let us say that the mandible is retruded.

The slope of the mandibular plane is rather flat, but within the range of normal. The slope of the Y axis is normal.

TABLE 3–3

		Children Mean S.D.
NP–Frankfort	83	89.4 ± 3.4
NAP	9	4.2 ± 5.4
SN–GoGn	30	32.3 ± 4.7
SGn–Frankfort	57	57.2 ± 3.3
SNA	80	80.8 ± 3.9
SNB	74.5	78.0 ± 3.1
Diff.	5.5	2.8
$\underline{1}$ to $\overline{1}$	158	130.4 ± 7.3
$\overline{1}$ to GoGn	81	93.5 ± 5.8
$\underline{1}$ to SN	92	103.5 ± 5.0

The angular value of SNA implies that the maxilla is normally positioned. The value for SNB is less than the mean, resulting in a large difference. Now the impression is strongly one of a retruded mandible.

The interincisal angle is much higher than normal. This is the result of the maxillary central incisors having a vertical inclination, while the mandibular central incisors are lingually inclined.

The interpretation of the skeletal and dental sections of the cephalometric analysis yields a diagnosis of a skeletal Class II occlusion resembling Class II division 2.

Cephalometrics, like other roentgenographic techniques, does have numerous shortcomings. However, with cephalometric roentgenograms there is an opportunity to apply considerable mathematical precision to the craniofacial complex.

There is always some uncertainty in the identification of landmarks, and some variations are introduced in tracing the landmarks. Some of this uncertainty arises because some landmarks are not sharply defined. The lack of definition is caused partly by the size of the source of the x-rays, not the focal spot of the tube, secondary radiation emitted by the patient, and blurring caused by the grain size of the film and of the intensifying screens. There is also loss of definition related to involuntary and voluntary movement of the patient while the radiograph is being exposed.

A point source of radiation, just as does a point source of light, will form a sharp shadow. Although the focal spots of most x-ray machines are quite small, these sources are not points, and as a result there will be some blurring.

During the interval that the head is exposed to radiation it will emit secondary radiation. The secondary radiation detracts from the quality of the radiograph by fogging the image. Secondary radiation is emitted in random directions. It can be filtered from the primary radiation by the placing of a grid between the head of the patient and the cassette holding the film.

Fine grain film and fine grain intensifying screens both require more radiation to effect a satisfactory exposure of the film. Usually a compromise is made by using a medium speed film and medium speed intensifying screens (larger grain size), despite some loss of sharpness, in order to reduce the exposure time.

A long exposure time contributes to blurring because fidgeting children have more time to move. However, even if the patient does not move voluntarily, the heartbeat causes involuntary movement.

A more detailed examination of some of the landmarks used in radiographic cephalometrics can further erode confidence.

The Frankfort horizontal plane is used because it is an approximation of the horizontal plane that the head of a person assumes when he is in the free-standing position. The points determining the plane are also approximations. The ear rods may not be in contact with the highest point of the auditory meatus, and orbitale is often difficult to identify on the film.

Nasion is a junction point on a sliding suture. It is on a bony surface that is undergoing growth into the postadolescent years. The location of nasion changes with time, not only anteroposteriorly but occasionally vertically as well.

Point A, supposedly a skeletal point, can change by lingual or labial movement of the roots of the incisors. In addition, accurate identification of the long axes of the roots of incisors is often difficult. Criticism can be given to the accuracy of most of the other landmarks, too.

The magnitudes of the mean values and the standard deviations of the various angles are determined by studies on children from the general population with satisfactory growth and occlusal relationships. Points to consider are: (1) how satisfactory occlusion was defined, (2) the size of the sample, and (3) the significance of age, sex and race.

This critique is not made to disparage radiographic cephalometrics as an aid in evaluating occlusal disharmonies but to encourage the dentist in the intelligent use of cephalometric analysis.

REFERENCES

Altemus, L. A.: Cephalofacial relationships. Angle Orthod., *38*:175, 1968.

Chan, G. K.: A cephalometric appraisal of the Chinese. Am. J. Orthod., *61*:279, 1972.

Downs, W. B.: Variations in facial relationships: their significance in treatment and prognosis. Am. J. Orthod., *34*:812, 1948.

Enlow, D. H.: Growth and architecture of the face. J.A.D.A., *82*:763, 1971.

Krogman, W. M.: Use of computers in orthodontic analysis and diagnosis: A symposium. Am. J. Orthod., *61*:219, 1972.

Moore, A. W.: Cephalometrics as a diagnostic tool. J.A.D.A., *82*:775, 1971.

4

Headgear

JOHN ORR

There are thousands of children with an early mixed dentition occlusal disharmony who do not receive orthodontic treatment because the practitioner has not been adequately trained in his predoctoral dental program to recognize, treat or refer these children for treatment. There are many more children who cannot afford to have treatment owing to the high cost of orthodontics.

With the greater demand for health care delivery that will develop in the future, it will become mandatory for the general dental practitioner to recognize and treat early occlusal disharmonies in the mixed dentition. In accordance with this concept this chapter on headgear therapy is written — to interest and teach the pedodontist and general dental practitioner how to use headgear therapy, in order to intercept uncomplicated Class II occlusal disharmonies and to regain arch space in Class I occlusal disharmonies when there has been some arch length loss owing to mesial migration of maxillary first molars.

Angle in 1887 stated that the "value of the occipital bandage is becoming more and more appreciated and is especially applicable in cases of maxillary protrusion." He employed it in many cases and found it more satisfactory than other appliances in use at this time.

Kingsley, Case and many other practitioners in the early 1800's described and recommended the use of headgear in orthodontic treatment. Early in 1900, Baker introduced the use of intermaxillary elastic force in which the maxillary arch was pitted against the mandibular arch. The Baker anchorage and the expansion of dental arches became popular at this time. Headgear lost its popularity until practitioners realized that a significant number of patients treated by expansion of the dental arches were subject to relapses. It became evident that teeth that were not supported by basal bone were not in a stable position.

Kloehn in 1947 rejuvenated extraoral treatment for Class II division 1 occlusal disharmonies and emphasized the value of cervical traction in restraining maxillary growth and at the same time allowing mandibular development in a downward and forward direction. Early treatment in the mixed dentition, utilizing headgear, was stressed by Kloehn to reduce treatment time and allow more stable occlusion. Allowing the Class II occlusal disharmony to progress into the permanent dentition makes treatment longer and more difficult and in large numbers of cases necessitates the extraction of teeth.

Premature loss of the maxillary second primary molars allows the mesial migration of the maxillary first permanent molars, resulting in a Class II occlusal relationship. The cervical strap and Kloehn face bow are particularly useful in moving the maxillary first permanent molars distally, regaining arch length and allowing the maxillary premolars to take their proper place in the arch.

There are innumerable types of face bows and cervical straps that are available to the profession. The discussion of headgear therapy in this chapter will describe the *Kloehn* type of headgear that has been found to be useful in intercepting Class II occlusal disharmonies with closed bites in the mixed dentition, and guiding first permanent molars that have drifted mesially owing to premature loss of maxillary primary second molars.

Class II occlusal disharmonies with open bites are more complicated and will not be discussed here. This type of occlusal disharmony is best treated by an orthodontist or dental practitioner who has had orthodontic training and experience.

THE FACE BOW (Figs. 4–1 to 4–4)

There are many opinions regarding the effectiveness of headgear therapy in Class II division 1 occlusal disharmonies. Headgear therapy

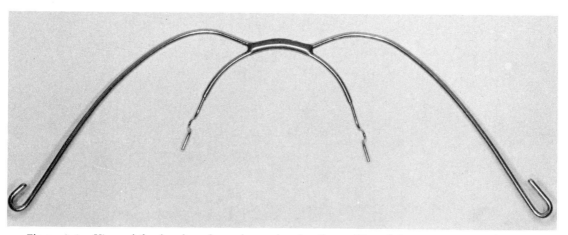

Figure 4–1. View of the face bow from above, showing the position of the outer arms in relation to the molar stops on the inner arms of the bow.

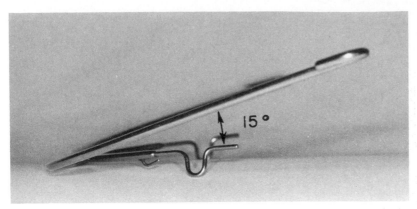

Figure 4–2. The side view of the face bow, showing the 15 degree angle that the outer arms have to the inner arms of the bow. The loop molar stops that prevent the bow from sliding any further distally through the buccal tubes are also apparent. Anterior to the molar stops on the inner arch are the anterior hooks, to which elastics are attached for the intrusion and retrusion of the anterior teeth.

may help move the maxillary molars distally but it is more effective in exerting a restraining influence on the forward growth of the maxilla. When maxillary growth is restrained with headgear therapy, mandibular growth may then progress to its fullest potential.

The majority of Class II division 1 occlusal disharmonies often have mandibular arches that are satisfactory in arch form, contact relationships, tooth size and incisors over basal bone. It becomes apparent that the greatest number of Class II division 1 occlusal disharmonies are disharmonies of jaw relationships.

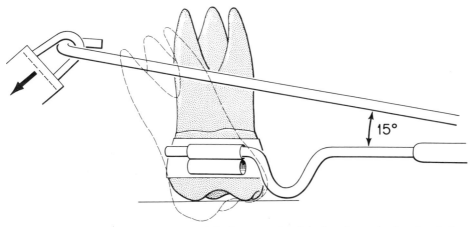

Figure 4–3. When the outer arms of the bow are placed so that they extend up in relation to the occlusal plane, the overall effect is the bodily distal movement of the upper molars.

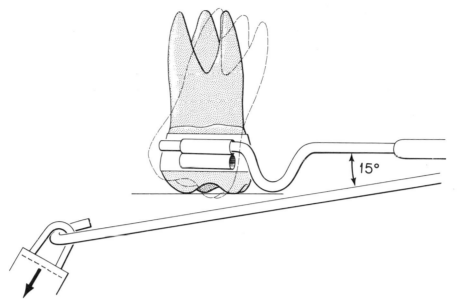

Figure 4–4. When the outer arms of the bow are placed so that they extend down in relation to the occlusal plane, the action of the cervical strap is to tip the molar in a distal direction.

Selection of Molar Bands for Headgear Therapy

Preformed bands may be used, preferably bands that have right and left orientation.

Preformed bands are carefully adapted to the maxillary first permanent molars. There are many commercially available bands that come in right and left types in various sizes.

If one prefers loop bands in stainless steel or precious metal, they may be purchased in four different sizes (manufactured by the Baker Company). I prefer the precious metal loop band because it is easier to work with and may readily be soldered with a nontarnishing gold solder. A band is selected that fits the maxillary molar so that there is only a slight opening of the small loop on the mesiobuccal cusp. The band is always placed on the tooth with the loop adjacent to the mesiobuccal cusp.

Seating of Bands for Headgear Therapy

Often, when the contacts are close, separation must be used to reduce pain and trauma in sealing and adapting the bands.

1. The band is placed on the tooth and with the aid of a beavertail band seater or a tongue blade the band is forced gently through the contact points (Fig. 4–6).

2. After the initial seating of the band more exact seating is carried out by having the patient bite the band into place with the aid of a tongue blade, and final seating and adaptation may then be accomplished with a

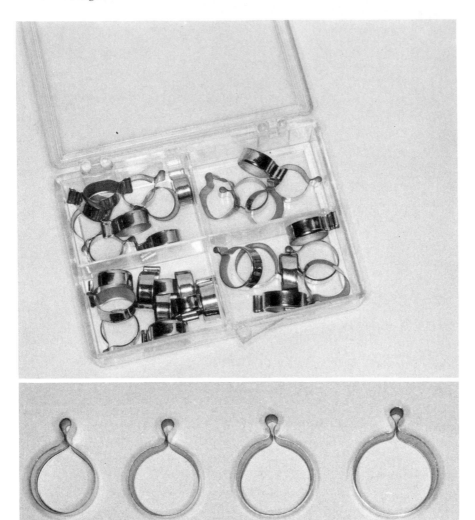

Figure 4–5. Loop bands come in four sizes and can be fitted to any molar. The advantage in using loop bands is that any molar may be fitted without carrying a large inventory of bands.

band pusher or any other instrument of choice (Fig. 4–7). When the band is seated properly on the tooth Howe pliers may be used to grasp the small loop adjacent to the mesiobuccal cusp, squeezing the loop, thus drawing the band material tightly around the tooth (Fig. 4–8).

3. After the right and left maxillary bands have been carefully adapted they are removed and solder is run into the small crevice in the loops that were pinched together (Fig. 4–9). The bands are then reseated on the teeth, and an alginate or silicone impression taken over the bands. After the impression is taken the bands are carefully removed from the maxillary molars with the band-removing pliers. The bands are then carefully seated in the impression and reinforced by sticky wax. It is suggested that a paper clip wire be imbedded and bent at right angles into the occlusal surface of the molar before pouring the stone cast (Fig. 4–10). This wire will reinforce the molar tooth and prevent the tooth from breaking loose from the rest of the cast when the model has been heated

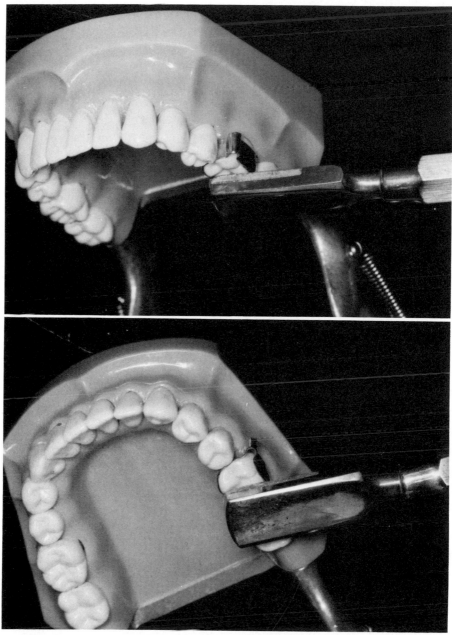

Figure 4–6. The band is started through the contact points by using a broad band seater with a soft tin insert to apply pressure over a large surface of the band. The occlusal edge of the band may be covered by the seater, and the band seater rocked back and forth to start the seating through the contacts.

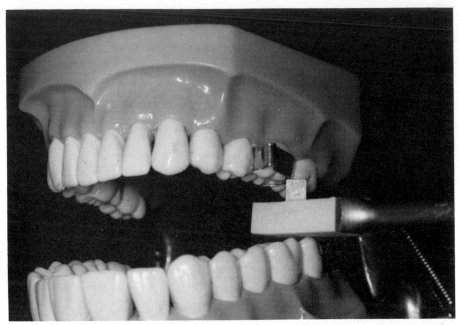

Figure 4–7. Further seating of the band is done by having the patient bite the band into place using one of the band seaters similar to the one shown. Hand seaters having serrated metal tips are also useful at this time to accomplish final seating of the band.

in the soldering operation. After the stone cast has been separated from the impression the ends of the paper clips may be ground level with the occlusal surface of the molars using a heatless stone (Fig. 4–11*A*). Figure 4–11*A* shows how the immediately separated stone cast would appear before the paper clip wires were cut down to the occlusal level with a heatless stone (Fig. 4–11*B*, *C*).

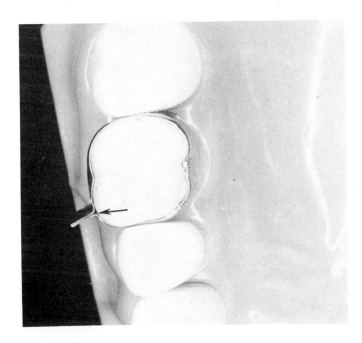

Figure 4–8. The pinched loop would appear as shown in this photograph after the band had been squeezed with Howe pliers.

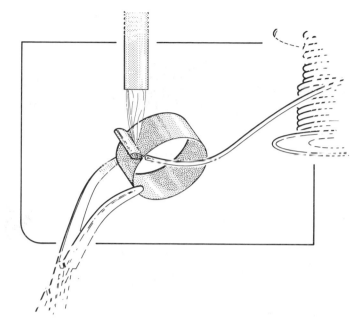

Figure 4–9. Silver solder is added to the inside of the band and allowed to fill the small pinched loop.

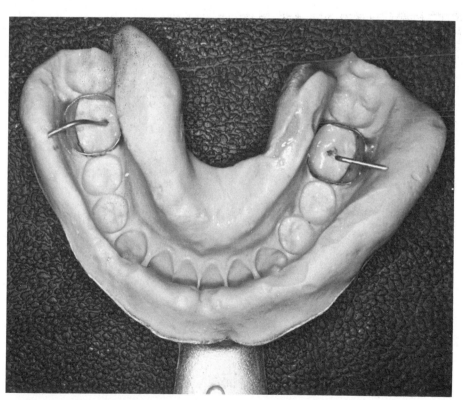

Figure 4–10. Paper clip wire is bent into the shape of an L and inserted into the impression of the occlusal surface of the molar and is inserted into the buccal extension of the impression to stabilize the wire when pouring the stone cast.

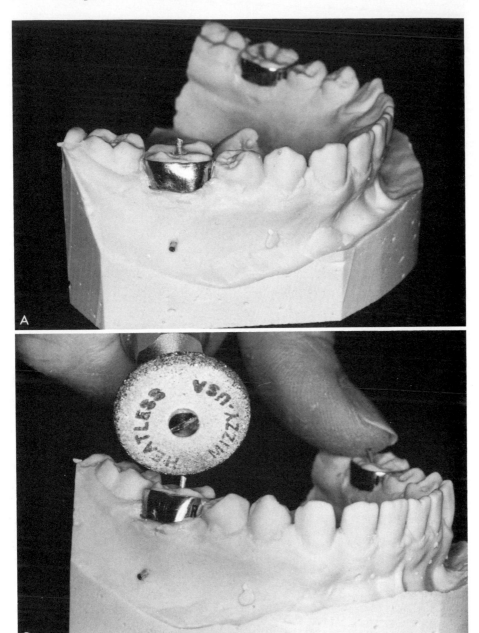

Figure 4–11

A, After the cast is poured, the cut ends of paper clip wire can be seen extending from the occlusal surface of the molar and from the buccal surface of the cast.

B, A heatless stone is used to grind the wire until it is even with the occlusal surface if the upper and lower casts need to be articulated.

Illustration continued on opposite page.

Next apply a liberal amount of silver solder to the buccal surface of the band (Fig. 4–12). The purpose of this solder is twofold: (1) to bond the double buccal tubes to the band, and (2) to make the band more rigid so that the extraoral force will not flex the band material and cause the cement seal to break. Molar bands do not become loose or require recementation as often as when welded double buccal tubes are used if

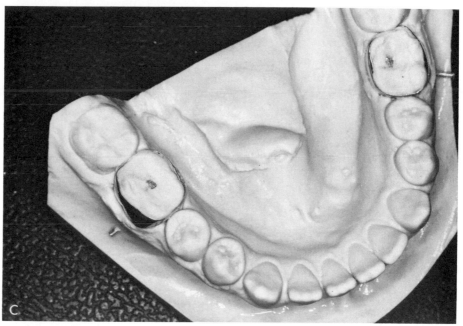

Figure 4–11 (*Continued*)

C, Occlusal appearance of the paper clip wire after being ground even with the occlusal surface. This wire prevents the stone molar from breaking off the cast when heat is applied to the band in the soldering procedures.

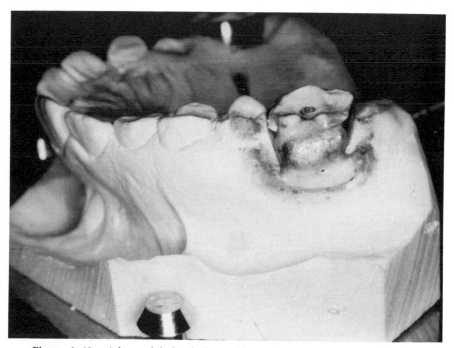

Figure 4–12. A large globule of silver solder is placed on the buccal surface of the molar band. This serves two purposes: (1) it adds rigidity to the molar band, and (2) it attaches the buccal tubing to the molar band.

the buccal tubes are soldered in this manner. The next laboratory procedure is to attach the double buccal tubes to the molar bands. This technique is the same whether the looped bands are used or whether preformed bands are used. Double buccal tubing is prepared by taking 12 in. lengths of 0.040 in. and 0.050 in. stainless steel tubing material and tack welding them together every 2 mm.

After the tubes are held together with the tact welds, a generous amount of silver solder is applied over the fluxed tubes to bond them together (Fig. 4–13). Two 12 in. lengths are made in this manner so that the buccal tubes can be accurately aligned in a manner that makes them meet at a point in front of the work model that lies in the midline.

The tubes are also soldered to the molar band so that the arch wire extending from the 0.040 in. buccal tube will approximate the gingival crest of the upper anterior teeth (Fig. 4–14*A*). This procedure will tend to depress the upper anterior teeth and will open the bite, which is usually necessary in a Class II division 1 occlusal disharmony. After the double buccal tubes are soldered to the molar bands, they are cut off with a separation disk until the tubing left on the molar band is about ¼ in. long. At this point it is time to adapt the face bow to the work model. A face bow having short outer arms is lipped to the outer bow at a 15 degree angle and anterior elastic hooks are fitted to the cast. The distance of the inner arch from the upper anterior teeth should be about ¼ in.

The inner arch should have about ¼ in. expansion on one side when the other end of the inner arch is in the opposite molar buccal tube (Fig. 4–15). This expansion of the molars keeps them from going into crossbite as they are moved distally into a wider portion of the dental arch.

The molar bands are now removed from the stone work model by

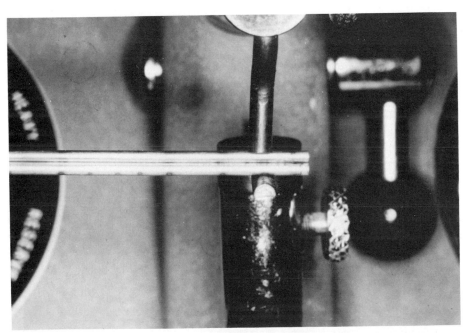

Figure 4–13

Tact welds are placed every 2 to 3 mm. along the 12 in. lengths of 0.040 in. and 0.050 in. buccal tubing. This photograph shows the two pieces of tubing between the electrodes of the spot welder.

heating the occlusal surface of the stone with an orthodontic blowtorch and immediately immersing the stone into water. The bands are then cleaned and polished for cementation in the mouth. When cementing the molar bands, it must be remembered that there is no lingual arch to help place the bands in the same position on the teeth as they were on the stone work model, and if they are not carried to exactly the same positions as on the work model, all efforts in aligning the buccal tubes on the model will be to no avail. To ensure the accurate cementation of the molar bands, aligning rods of 0.040 in. wire are used in the 0.040 in. buccal tubes during the cementation and are allowed to extend from the patient's mouth (Fig. 4–16).

By using these rods, the bands can be carried to positions that allow the aligning rods to meet at a point in the midline and in the same horizontal plane (Fig. 4–17). Four preformed anterior bands having wide Siamese edgewise brackets are cemented on the upper incisor teeth. These devices serve two purposes: (1) the brackets hold the arch wire in place, and (2) the incisal wings of the edgewise bracket serve as a catch for the anterior elastic on the face bow so that the elastic will tend to include these teeth as they are retracted. Reduction of the protrusion of the upper incisors can be started with this elastic even before the arch wire is placed. Many times it is best to wait a month or two before placing the arch wire, after better bracket alignment has been obtained from the pressure exerted by the anterior elastic.

By placing the anterior elastic (usually a ³⁄₄ in. light latex) incisally to the brackets, intrusive force is generated which tends to depress the incisors into their sockets and thus opens the bite (Fig. 4–18).

At later appointments, as the upper molars assume a Class I relationship, an arch wire is constructed using 0.0355 in. end section tubing on which Class II hooks have been placed by the manufacturer (Fig. 4–19). The wire used for the anterior section of the arch will vary according to whether the upper incisors are rotated or whether they are out of alignment labiolingually. If bracket engagement cannot easily be obtained, a multistranded wire is used in the end section tubes so that the incisors can be gently rotated or moved labiolingually. This wire is made by several manufacturers and usually consists of three or four strands of wire twisted together. After bracket engagement is obtained, the arch is remade using 0.016 in. Australian wire in the end section tubing. The easiest way to lock the multistrand wire or Australian wire in the end section is by using the "Rocky Mountain Ruff" pliers to crimp the end section tubing.

The next step in treatment is to place the patient on Class II elastics to help in the correction of the anterior protrusion (Fig. 4–20). Since the headgear treatment is being limited to patients who have good lower arches, a corrective appliance is not necessary in the lower arch; only an anchorage appliance is needed. A soldered lower lingual arch can usually be used for this purpose. The construction of the work model is exactly the same as for the upper model. From the work model a 0.036 in. steel blue Elgiloy stainless steel lingual arch is constructed to fit accurately against the lower anterior teeth at the gingival margin, and is soldered to the molar bands with silver solder. On the buccal surface of the molar

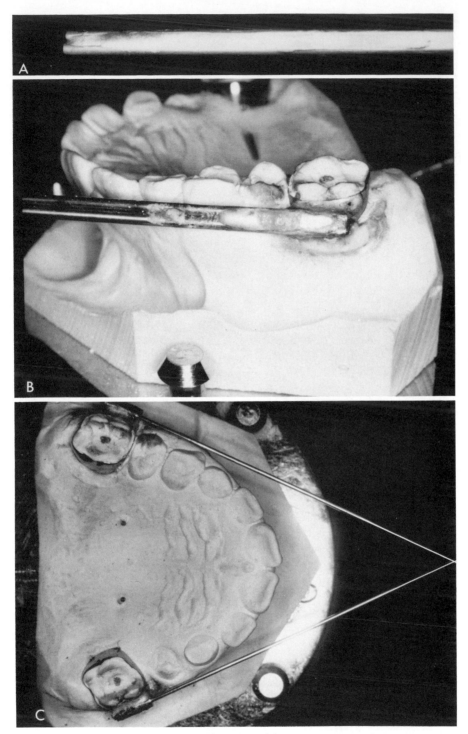

Figure 4–14

A, After welding, silver solder is allowed to flow into the crevice between the two pieces of tubing.

B, The tubing is then placed in the proper position with the molar band, and the blowtorch is applied to bond the tubes to the band.

C, The buccal tubes are placed so that when 0.040 in. aligning rods are placed in the 0.040 in. buccal tubes, they cross at a point in the midline anterior to the incisors.

Illustration continued on opposite page.

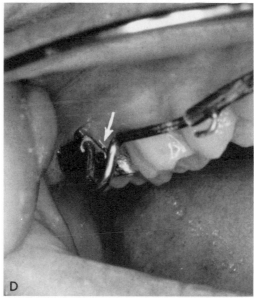

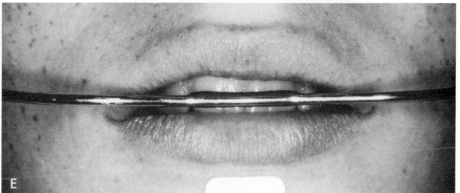

Figure 4–14 (*Continued*)

D, Position of the inner arm of the face bow when placed into the buccal tube in the mouth.

E, The face bow should lie passively between the upper and lower lips.

F, That size face bow is selected which will stand out from the upper anterior teeth about ¼ in. when the bow is placed into the buccal tubes.

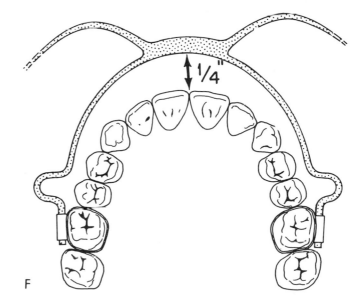

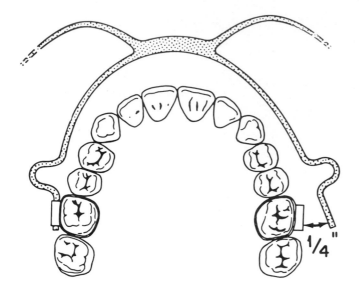

Figure 4–15

About ¼ in. of expansion is provided in the inner bow to keep the molars moving buccally as they move distally. If this is not done, the upper molar will gradually go into a crossbite.

bands 0.030 in. hooks are soldered, onto which the Class II elastics are attached.

Class II elastics exerting a force of 2 to 3 ounces of pressure as measured on a Dontrix gauge are worn only when the headgear is not in place (Fig. 4–21); thus the lower arch is not subjected to the continuous detrimental effect of wearing the Class II elastics for a 24 hour period.

Pressures Used in Extraoral Force

The amount of extraoral force placed on the headgear depends on whether one prefers tooth movement or whether an orthopedic force is to be placed on the maxilla. If one wants to move the first molars distally, the patient should be placed on about 8 ounces of pressure as measured on the Dontrix scale (Fig. 4–21) at the first appointment. After the first month the pressure can be increased to between 12 and 16 ounces. Practitioners who apply orthopedic forces to the maxilla in order to actually reposition the whole maxillary arch will use forces of 1 to 2 pounds. A convenient method of measuring these heavy orthopedic forces is to attach to the neck strap a fisherman's scale that reads in pounds.

The patient undergoing headgear therapy needs to wear the appliance for a minimum of 14 hours of each 24 hour period. These 14 hours do not have to be continuous, but the patient should keep an accurate record each day in writing to be certain the 14 hours are attained. We have found it best to give the child a mimeographed form to use for this purpose, which will show at a glance the total number of hours attained for each day. If for some reason the full 14 hours were not attained in one day, the difference should be made up so that at the end of the week there is a total of at least 98 hours.

(Text continued on page 61.)

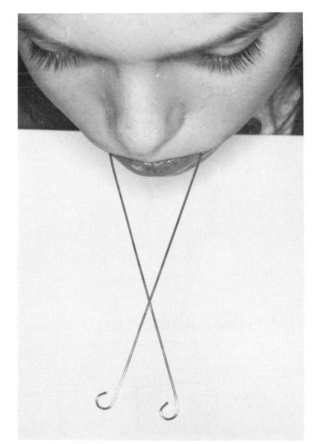

Figure 4–16. Aligning rods (0.040 in.) are placed in the 0.040 in. buccal tubes when cementing the molar bands to make sure they are cemented in exactly the same position they occupied on the work cast. These rods are allowed to extend out of the mouth while the bands are being cemented into place.

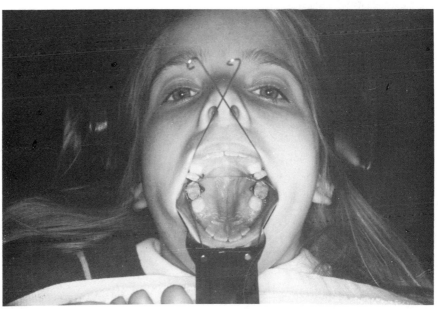

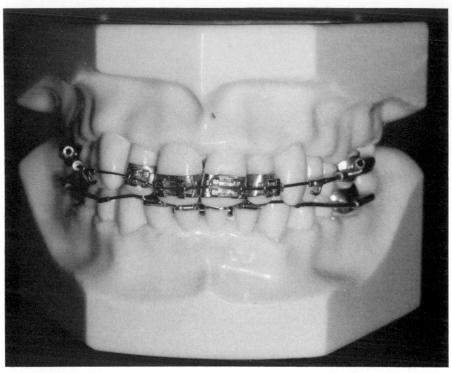

Figure 4–17. Siamese edgewise brackets with multistranded light wire tied in place. (G.A.C. wildcat wire, Unitek twist-flex or American Orthodontic twist wire may be used.) The 0.050 buccal tube for the headgear can be seen gingivally to the arch wire.

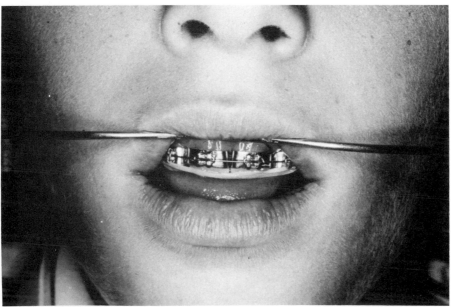

Figure 4–18. The intra-oral photograph shows the anterior elastic attached to the face bow hooks and lying gingivally to the Siamese brackets, which will tend to intrude the incisors while reducing the protrusion.

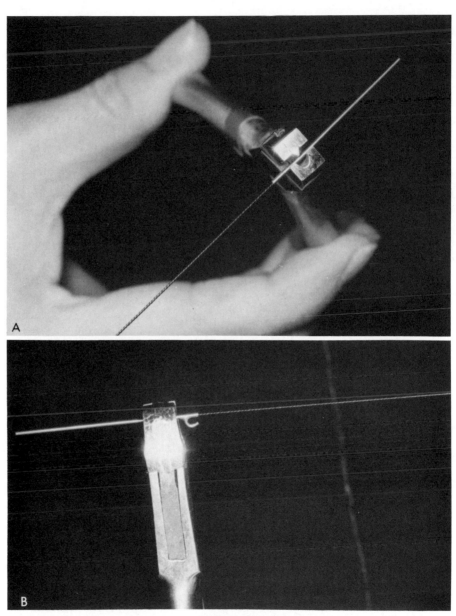

Figure 4–19

A, Rocky Mountain Ruff pliers holding end section tubing before squeezing pliers to crimp end section.

B, Note hook on end section for Class II elastics.

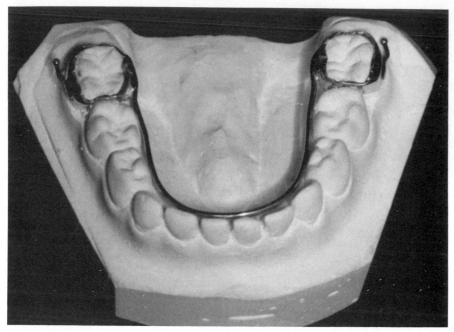

Figure 4–20. Lower lingual arch used for anchorage against Class II elastics. The 0.036 in. steel lingual must fit tightly against the cingulum of the lower anterior teeth. The hooks on the buccal surface of the molar bands are for engagement of the elastics.

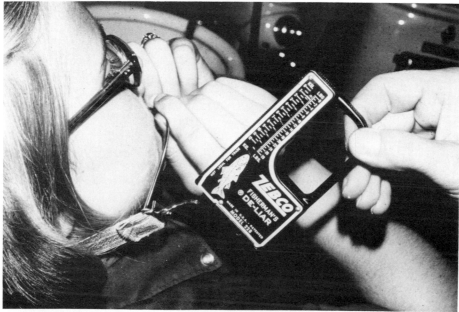

Figure 4–21. A fisherman's scale may be used for measuring the force placed on the cervical strap.

REFERENCES

Angle, E. H.: New system of regulation and retention. Dent. Reg., *41*:597–603, 1887.

Begg, P. R., and Kesling, P. C.: Begg Orthodontic Theory and Technique. 2nd Ed. Philadelphia, W. B. Saunders Co., 1971.

Blueher, W. A.: Cephalometric analysis of treatment with cervical anchorage. Angle Orthod., *29*:45–53, 1959.

Brickbauer, G. P.: Preventive and interceptive orthodontics for the growing child. Int. J. Orthod., *10*:47–51, 1972.

Brock, W. C.: The principle of coil splinting traction applied to cervical strap therapy. Am. J. Orthod., *46*:43–45, 1960.

Chaconas, S. J.: Malocclusions: Incipient or transient? Am. Soc. Preventive Dent., July-August 1972, p. 36.

DeCastro, N.: The challenge of Class II division 1 malocclusion. Am. J. Orthod., *46*:829–833, 1960.

Epstein, W. N.: Analysis of changes in molar relationships by means of extraoral anchorage (headcap) in treatment of malocclusion. Angle Orthod., *18*:63–69, 1948.

Gould, I. E.: Mechanical principles in extraoral anchorage. Am. J. Orthod., *43*:319–333, 1957.

Graber, T. M.: Extraoral force—facts and fallacies. Am. J. Orthod., *41*:262–278, 1955.

Graber, T. M.: Orthodontics: Principles and Practice. 3rd Ed. Philadelphia, W. B. Saunders Co., 1972.

Graber, T. M., and Swain, B. F. (Eds.): Current Orthodontic Concepts and Techniques. Vol. II. 2nd Ed., Philadelphia, W. B. Saunders Co., 1975.

Gregorak, W.: Eruption path of permanent maxillary molars in Class II division 1 malocclusion using headgear. Am. J. Orthod., *48*:367–381, 1962.

Haack, D. C.: The mechanics of centric and eccentric cervical traction. Am. J. Orthod., *44*:346–357, 1958.

Hanes, R. A.: Boney profile changes resulting from cervical traction compared with those resulting from intermaxillary elastics. Am. J. Orthod., *45*:353–364, 1959.

Kanter, F.: Mandibular anchorage and extraoral force. Am. J. Orthod., *42*:194–208, 1956.

King, E. W.: Cervical anchorage in Class II division 1 treatment—a cephalometric appraisal. Angle Orthod., *17*:98–103, 1947.

Klein, P. L.: An evaluation of cervical traction on the maxilla and the first permanent molars. Angle Orthod., *27*:61–68, 1957.

Kloehn, S. J.: A new approach to the analysis and treatment in mixed dentition. Am. J. Orthod., *39*:161–186, 1953.

Kloehn, S. J.: Guiding alveolar growth and eruption of teeth to reduce treatment time and produce a more balanced denture and face. Angle Orthod., *17*:10–33, 1947.

Kloehn, S. J.: Mixed dentition treatment. Angle Orthod., *20*:75–96, 1950.

Mollin, A. D.: Universal Light Arch Technique. New York, Leo L. Bruder, 1966.

Moss, L.: Extraoral force in modern orthodontics. Int. J. Orthod., *8*:154–163, 1970.

Newcomb, M. R.: Some observations on extra-oral treatment. Angle Orthod., *28*:131–148, 1958.

Poulton, D. R.: Changes in Class II malocclusions with and without occipital headgear therapy. Angle Orthod., *29*:232–250, 1959.

Poulton, D. R.: A three year survey of Class II malocclusions with and without headgear therapy. Angle Orthod., *34*:181–193, 1964.

Poulton, D. R.: The influence of extra-oral traction. Am. J. Orthod., *53*:8–18, 1967.

Sandusky, W. C.: Cephalometric evaluation of the effects of the Kloehn type of cervical traction used as an auxiliary with the edgewise mechanism following Tweed's principles for correction of Class II division 1 malocclusion. Am. J. Orthod., *51*:262–287, 1955.

Tweed, C. H.: Clinical Orthodontics. St. Louis, C. V. Mosby Co., 1966.

Weber, N. F.: Prophylactic orthodontics. Am. J. Orthod., *35*:611–635, 1949.

5

The Primary Dentition

Irregularities of the primary dentition are often harbingers of disorders of the developing dentition. Treatment of these irregularities as soon as they are recognized will in many instances prevent or reduce the severity of an occlusal disharmony.

It is most essential to examine the primary dentition carefully, utilizing roentgenograms (Panorex if possible), plaster casts and cephalometric x-rays when indicated. A careful examination of both hard and soft tissues as well as observation of the jaws closed in centric relationship is essential for identifying occlusal disharmonies. In addition to a careful dental examination the practitioner should engage the child in conversation to observe any deviations in speech, presence of oral habits and the swallowing habits of the child. The practitioner should also examine the child's fingers for calluses, which are often associated with oral habits.

The primary teeth begin to develop in embryogenesis, at approximately 33 days in utero. From this period to the postnatal age of 3 to 3½ years odontogenesis takes place and in the absence of adverse prenatal and postnatal influences the preschool child should have a full complement of primary teeth.

OCCLUSAL RELATIONSHIPS

The primary teeth vary in size, morphology, spacing and occlusal relationships (Fig. 5–1).

The primary dental arches are arranged in either a spaced or a closed relationship. Spaces may be observed between all teeth or between specific groups of teeth. In the spaced arch, primate spaces between the primary maxillary lateral incisor and the primary canine may be observed.

In the mandible, primate spaces may be found between the mandibular primary canines and the mandibular primary molars. The closed primary arches are more constricted than the spaced arches. Both the spaced and closed primary dentitions are congenital, not developmental,

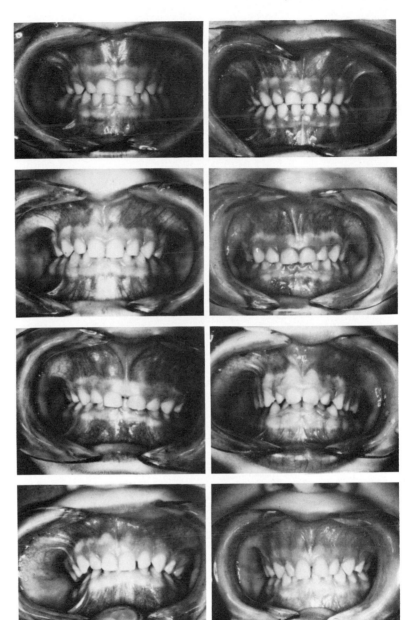

Figure 5–1. Variation of primary teeth (see text.)

with the exception of spacing between the first and second primary molars, which usually close between the ages of $2\frac{1}{2}$ and $3\frac{1}{2}$ years.

Classification of Occlusal Relationships

The occlusal relationships of the primary arches may be classified according to the relationships of the maxillary and mandibular second primary molars, as well as the occlusal relationships of the primary canines. the following is a modification of the Angle occlusal relationship in the primary dentition.

    I. Class Ia. Neutroclusion
       Class Ib. Neutroclusion
   II. Class II. Distoclusion
 III. Class III. Mesioclusion

CLASS IA. NEUTROCLUSION (SPACED)

In class Ia neutroclusion the distal surface of the mandibular primary second molar is mesial to the distal surface of the maxillary primary second molar. In the primary spaced arch the maxillary canine occludes in the primate space between the mandibular canine and first molar (Fig. 5–2).

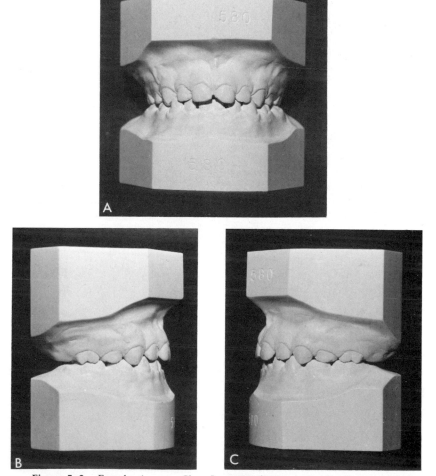

Figure 5–2. Female, 4 years. Class Ia neutroclusion (spaced) (*A*). Note maxillary canine occluding into primate space between mandibular canine and first molar (*B*) and mesial relationship of mandibular molar to maxillary molar (*C*).

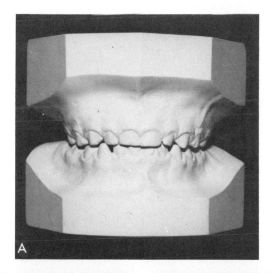

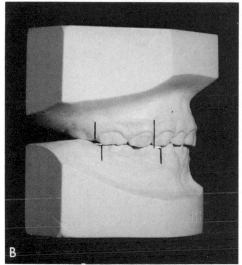
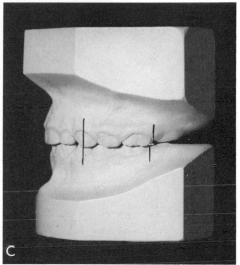

Figure 5–3. Male, 4 years. Class Ib neutroclusion (*A*). Note maxillary canine occluding into primate space and mesial relationship of mandibular molar to maxillary molar (*B*). *C*, End-to-end relationship of primary canines and vertical relationship of primary second molars.

CLASS IB. NEUTROCLUSION (NON-SPACED)

In class Ib neutroclusion, the distal surfaces of the mandibular primary second molar and the maxillary second molar are in the same vertical plane, and the canine interlock is absent since there is no primate space between the mandibular canine and mandibular first primary molar. The canines usually are in an end-to-end relationship. This type of occlusion is often observed when the primary teeth are not spaced (Fig. 5–3).

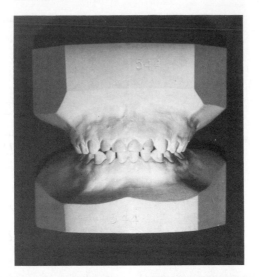

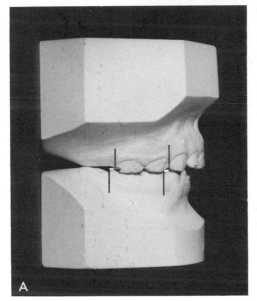

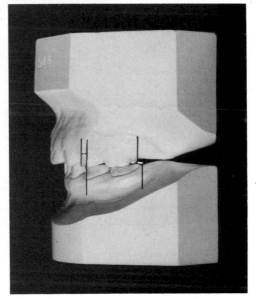

Figure 5–4

A, Male, 4 years. Class II distoclusion. Note distal relationship of mandibular molars to maxillary molars.

Illustration continued on opposite page

CLASS II. DISTOCLUSION

In Class II distoclusion the distal surfaces of the mandibular molars are distal to the distal surfaces of the maxillary molars, and there is an end-to-end occlusion of the canines. In some cases the distoclusion involves the teeth alone, and in others there is an actual distal relationship involves the teeth alone, and in others there is an actual distal relationship to the mandible and the maxilla (Fig. 5–4A). A cephalometric roentgenogram will differentiate between distoclusal relationships of the teeth and an actual distal relationship of the mandible to the maxilla (Fig. 5–4B).

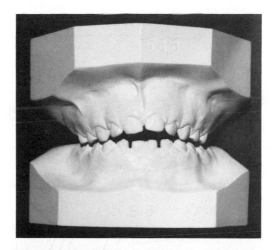

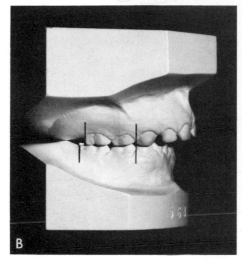
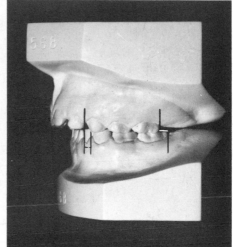

Figure 5-4 *Continued.* B, Male, 3½ years. Class II distoclusion. Note open bite resulting from oral habit and distal relationship of mandibular molars to maxillary molars.

CLASS III. MESIOCLUSION

The distal surfaces of the mandibular second molars are in a marked mesial relationship to the distal surfaces of the maxillary second molars, and the mandibular canines are in a mesial relationship to the maxillary canines. The mandibular incisors are labial to the maxillary incisors. The majority of mesioclusions in the primary dentition are the result of an anterior crossbite. Occasionally a true mesioclusion or prognathism may be observed in the primary dentition. The relationship can be confirmed only with a cephalometric roentgenogram (Fig. 5-5).

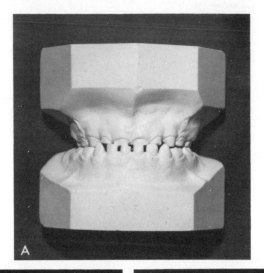

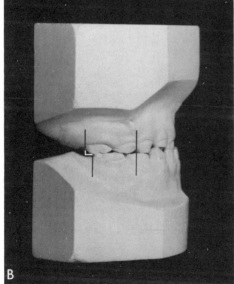
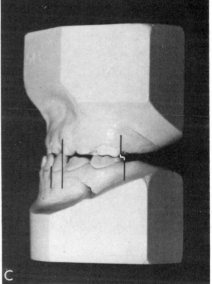

Figure 5–5. Female, 4½ years. Class III mesioclusion. Note mesial relationship of maxillary incisors to mandibular incisors and mesial relationship of maxillary molars to mandibular molars. (Courtesy of Dr. Leonard J. Carapezza, Wayland, Massachusetts.)

Variations in Occlusal Relationships

In the primary dentition, spacing between the incisors and primate spaces between primary canines and laterals, in both the maxilla and the mandible, vary in their occurrence and in size. The molar relationships in Class I occlusion also vary, and sometimes primary dentition may have a Class Ia relationship on one side and a Class Ib on the other side.

The same variations may be found in primary canine relationships, in which there may be an interlock on one side and an end-to-end relationship on the opposite side. These variations are found in the primary dentition, and a true Class Ia or Class Ib neutroclusion, as described in the text, is rarely observed. The modification of Angle's classification of the primary dentition should be used only as a guide to assess Class I occlusal relationships. These types of occlusal relationships should be considered satisfactory. In Class II relationships, the mandibular second molars may be distal by half a tooth or more to the maxillary molars, and the canine relationships may vary in their end-to-end occlusal relationships.

OCCLUSAL DISHARMONIES

There is a scarcity of reliable information on the incidence of occlusal disharmonies in the primary dentition. In 1956, 491 Brookline, Massachusetts, preschool children with the average age of 4.2 years were examined for the distribution of occlusal disharmonies, according to Angle's classification. Of these, 89.5 per cent were determined to be Class I jaw relationships; 10 per cent were Class II relationships; and 0.7 per cent were Class III relationships. It was found that a high percentage of the children (71 per cent) had no anterior spacing of the primary maxillary incisors. It has been stated that when there is no spacing of the anterior teeth in the primary dentition, the intercanine space development is greater than that found in children who have spacing. These findings have never been confirmed by longitudinal growth studies, and it is suggested that children who have no spacing in the anterior primary teeth be placed under observation, since this condition may lead to Class I irregularities in the permanent dentition.

Class II Relationships

True Class II occlusal disharmonies are found in the primary dentition in a small percentage of cases. Incidence may vary from 1 to 10 per cent and depends upon adverse prenatal influences, nutrition, genetic factors, geographic location and ethnic background of the population. The true Class II occlusal disharmonies in the primary dentition may be accurately confirmed with cephalometric x-rays.

Class III Relationships

The majority of Class III relationships observed in the primary dentition are anterior crossbites. True Class III relationships are rare in normal children, but are often found in children with congenital defects such as Down's syndrome, cerebral gigantism, Apert's syndrome, and cleidocranial dysostosis, and in families in which prognathism is an autosomal dominant characteristic.

Posterior Crossbite

The most frequent occlusal disharmony in the primary dentition is the posterior crossbite. The majority of posterior crossbites found in the primary dentition are environmental or functional in origin. There are, however, a very small number of skeletal crossbites that do occur. They are the result of a disharmonic development of either the maxilla or the mandible that manifests itself in a gross disharmony of the anterior or posterior occlusion. Skeletal crossbites may be unilateral or bilateral and are very difficult to treat. Although they are found occasionally in normal children, they are frequently observed in children with cleft lip and cleft palate, and in the following congenital disorders: Apert's syndrome, Crouzon's syndrome, Pfeiffer's syndrome, and achondroplasia.

It is suggested that the pediatric dentist or practitioner treat the skeletal crossbite early, provided that he has had orthodontic training, or that he refer the patient to an orthodontist for consultation, observation and treatment.

CLASSIFICATION

Posterior crossbites occur as follows:
1. Unilateral or bilateral linguoversion of mandibular molars to maxillary molars.
2. Unilateral or bilateral labioversion of mandibular molars.
3. Unilateral or bilateral linguoversion of maxillary molars to mandibular molars.
4. Maxillary molars in extreme labioversion to mandibular molars. (See Chapter 1.)

Posterior crossbites occur in the same order as the above classification in the mixed and permanent dentitions.

TREATMENT

All posterior crossbites should be treated as early as possible and the teeth placed in their proper occlusal relationships. Unilateral posterior crossbites very often lead to asymmetry of the occlusion, placing the midline in an abnormal position, and in accentuated cases there may be a deviation to the right or left, causing a facial asymmetry.

It is sometimes difficult to treat the very young child (ages 3 to 4 years) with posterior crossbite and it is advisable to wait until the child is 5 to 6 years of age before initiating treatment. Posterior crossbites may be treated with: (1) cross-elastics, (2) removable split plates, or (3) fixed expansion split plates, in which the molar bands are cemented onto the posterior teeth and an expansion screw is utilized.

1. Cross-elastics

Molar bands with labial or lingual buttons are adapted to teeth that are in crossbite; buttons are placed on either the labial or the lingual aspect of the band, depending on the type of crossbite. (See Chapter 1.) Careful instructions for wearing elastics should be given to the parents and patient (see *Instructions for Wearing Elastics.* See Chapter 1).

2. Removable Split Appliance

The removable split plate is an adaptation of the Hawley appliance with a labial arch wire, an expansion screw and an Adams or Arrow clasp.

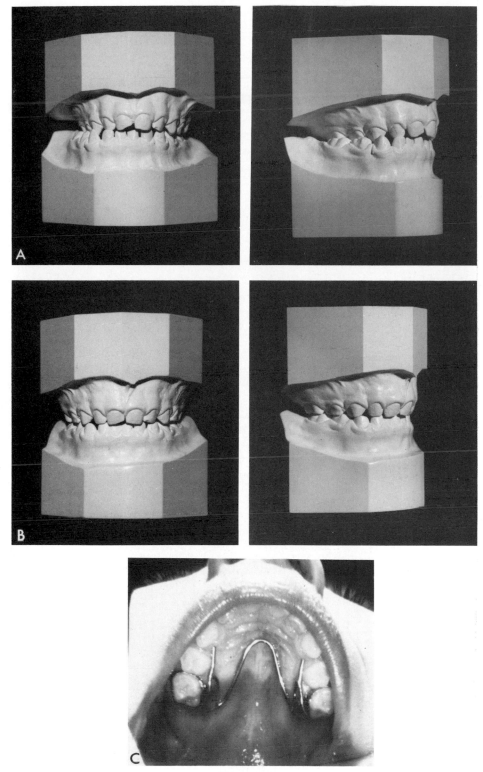

Figure 5–6

A, Unilateral crossbite involving maxillary lateral canine and primary molars before treatment.

B, After approximately 5 months of treatment with Porter expansion appliance.

C, Palatal view of Porter appliance.

The Adams or Arrow clasp engages the embrasures of the teeth and gives the appliance much more stability.

The practitioner must exercise extreme care in selecting young children for removable appliance therapy. Only a small percentage of young children may be expected to cooperate in wearing a removable appliance.

3. Fixed Expansion Appliance

An effective fixed appliance for treatment of posterior crossbites is a fixed appliance utilizing the Porter expansion arch or a Coffin spring (Figs. 5–6 and 5–7).

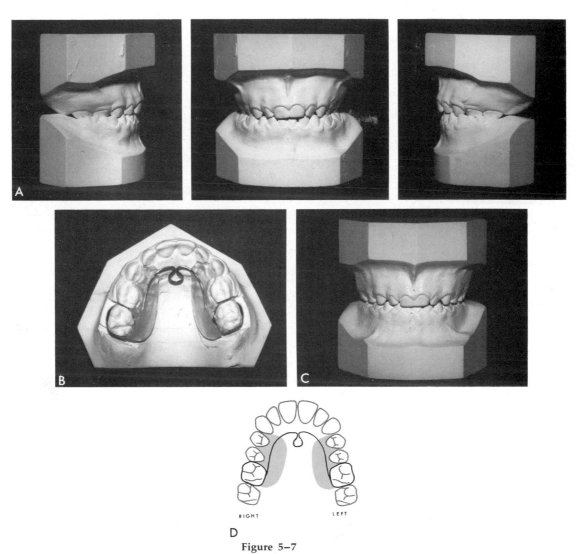

Figure 5–7

A, Bilateral posterior crossbite involving right and left first and second primary molars, canines and laterals.
B, Palatal view of fixed Coffin spring appliance.
C, Casts showing correction of bilateral crossbite.
D, Prescription for appliance: Maxillary fixed appliance with bands on maxillary primary second molars, acrylic extending from distal surface of primary second molars to distal surface of primary laterals.
(Courtesy of Dr. Mario Tobias, Mexico City, Mexico.)

Anterior Crossbite

Anterior crossbites occur less frequently than posterior cross bites and are sometimes improperly classified as Class III occlusal relationships.

TREATMENT

Anterior cross bites may be corrected by utilizing an inclined plane on the maxillary incisors, or an inclined plane made of acrylic is cemented on the mandibular teeth so that the maxillary teeth in linguoversion strike the inclined plane and in this way move the maxillary teeth into a satisfactory occlusal relationship (Fig. 5–8).

Another effective method for treating pseudo-Class III relationships is to band the maxillary second primary molars and the four maxillary in-

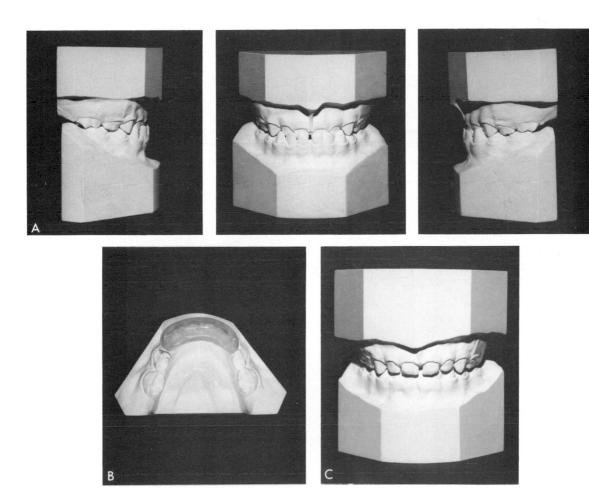

Figure 5–8

A, Frontal and lateral views of a pseudo Class III occlusal disharmony (anterior crossbite).
B, Acrylic inclined plane cemented on mandibular incisors and canines.
C, Casts showing correction of anterior crossbite.
(Courtesy of Dr. Leonard J. Carapezza, Wayland, Massachusetts.)

cisors utilizing a light wire or twin arch labial arch wire ligation. After the locked incisors are brought into the maxillary arch curve the labial arch wire may be left in place for a period of time to stabilize the teeth.

ORAL HABITS

THUMB SUCKING

Oral habits in infancy are learned and may be considered normal. Some infants are fascinated by their fingers and thumbs in early life and suck on them when irritable or hungry.

Epidemiological reports from various countries have shown that thumb and finger sucking occurs in approximately 20 per cent of the children examined. When an oral habit persists it may cause protrusion of the maxillary incisors with an open bite. In some cases sucking the thumb may exert pressure against the mandibular incisors and may cause linguoversion of these teeth.

There are innumerable appliances for the treatment and correction of the open bite and protrusion of the primary central incisors caused by thumb sucking. One of the most effective appliances for the treatment of open bites caused by a thumb sucking habit is the palatal crib. It may be used as either a fixed or removable appliance (Fig. 5–9). Cooperative children will wear removable appliances. Those less cooperative are treated best with a fixed appliance. Occasionally a plastic vestibular screen may be used for the improvement of nasal breathing and the breaking of a thumb sucking habit. Success in using a removable appliance depends on the following:

1. Gaining the full confidence of the child.

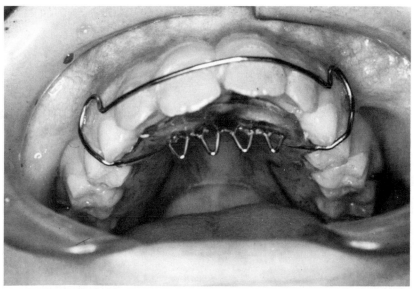

Figure 5–9. Removable appliance with palatal crib for controlling thumb sucking. (See Figure 7–10.)

2. The practitioner's ability to explain the benefits of the appliance in a simple and effective manner so that the child understands his responsibility in wearing the appliance for breaking the habit. The child may also be told that there will be a marked improvement in his facial appearance and his teeth will be brought into line.

Children who are conscientious about wearing removable appliances respond favorably in a short period of time.

A fixed palatal crib is the treatment of choice with most young children. Bands or stainless steel crowns may be used. A 0.040 in. stainless steel wire is utilized for soldering or welding the prongs onto the palatal crib. The loops or prongs are bent palatally so that the prongs are slightly posterior to the maxillary incisors.

TONGUE THRUSTING

It has been well established that tongue habits increase the overjet by moving the maxillary anterior teeth upward and forward, resulting in an open bite. There are innumerable causes of tongue thrusting, and this condition should be carefully evaluated before treatment is instituted. It is wise to consult a pediatrician and a speech therapist to determine whether speech therapy is indicated in conjunction with oral therapy.

One of the most effective appliances for controlling tongue thrusting is the palatal crib of either acrylic or metal (Fig. 5–10). The palatal crib may be removable or fixed, depending upon the maturity and cooperation of the patient. The removable palatal crib is effective when the sugarless wafer and tongue exercises are seriously performed by the patient. (See Chapter 1, Figure 1–10*A* and *B*.)

ANKYLOGLOSSIA

When a lingual frenum is observed associated with a speech impediment or restricted tongue movement, it should be excised. The lingual frenum, unlike the labial frenum, is not influenced by the eruption of the permanent teeth and should be removed at the discretion of the practitioner (Fig. 5–11).

ANOMALIES

SUPERNUMERARY TEETH

Supernumerary teeth are quite rare in the primary dentition. They vary in their morphology and may appear as an additional maxillary or mandibular incisor. The most frequent type of supernumerary tooth is the mesiodens. It occurs most frequently in the maxillary incisor region and contributes to disturbances in the eruption of the permanent maxillary incisors. Reports from Lind on 1717 Swedish children showed an incidence of mesiodens of 3 per cent in boys and 1.3 per cent in girls.

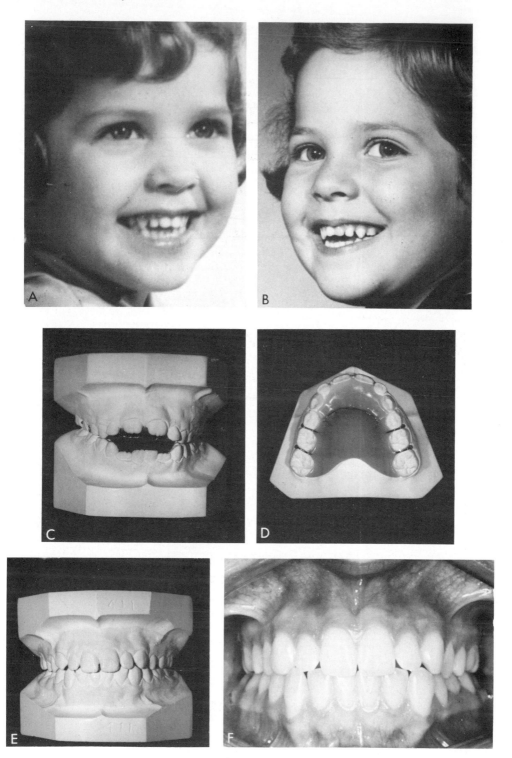

Figure 5–10

A, J. C., age 4. Note open bite owing to tongue habit.

B, J. C., age 5. Note increase in open bite from persistence of tongue habit.

C, Note further increase of open bite. Front view of open bite and removable appliance in place at age 7.

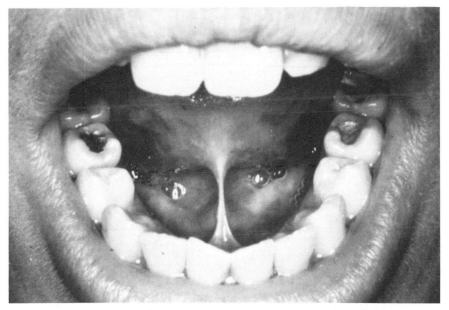

Figure 5–11. Lingual frenum (not associated with a speech impediment or restricted tongue movement).

Hüsgen reported an incidence of 3.4 per cent in 1000 German children. Menczer (1955), in a study of 2209 preschool children in Hartford, Connecticut, found only 11 dental anomalies. Of these, five were supernumerary teeth, four occurring as maxillary incisors and one occurring as a mandibular incisor (Fig. 5–12).

DIASTEMAS

Spacing between the primary central incisors is not uncommon. In young children this spacing may be physiological. Frequently in diastemas between the primary central incisors a large fibrous labial frenum may be observed. Although an abnormally enlarged frenum may appear to be a factor in the occurrence of a diastema, it is doubtful that it is of primary etiological significance. Some families have a familial pattern of diastemas, and it is wise to examine both the parents and the siblings of the child with the diastema (see Figure 5–13). A radiograph of the maxillary incisor region will show various bone patterns in the midline of the maxilla capable of causing diastemas. When these abnormal bone patterns are found to exist it is wise to alert the parents to the possibility of a diastema occur-

---

D, Appliance on model showing racklike fence positioned on palatal surface to confine tongue from striking lingual surfaces of maxillary and mandibular incisors. Rack wire soldered strips are 0.002 × 0.015 in. Ball clasps between embrasures are 01.S.028. Labial bow may be used in some cases and may be constructed of 0.030 in. wire. (In addition to wearing the appliance patient had a moderate amount of speech therapy).

E, Models of same patient at age 12.

F, Patient at age 17. Note satisfactory occlusal relationship after having worn a removable habit reminder for approximately 1 year and receiving a moderate amount of speech therapy at 7 years of age.

See illustration on opposite page.

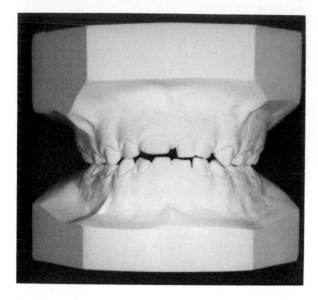

Figure 5–12. Fused primary central and lateral in the primary dentition.

ring in the permanent dentition. Frenectomy in the primary dentition is contraindicated since, in many cases, the height of the labial frenum becomes reduced with the vertical growth and development of the anterior part of the maxilla.

ANKYLOSIS

When a primary tooth ceases to erupt properly and the cementum becomes fused to the alveolar bone, the primary tooth assumes a position in the dental arch that is below the occlusal plane of the remaining teeth (Fig. 5–14). With the physiological growth and development of the dentition and the continuous eruption of the remaining unaffected primary teeth, the ankylosed tooth becomes further submerged in the alveolar bone, and in some instances ankylosed teeth have been found deep in the maxilla and the mandible, causing mesial and distal drifting of the permanent teeth and creating a serious orthodontic problem. The teeth most frequently found ankylosed are the first and second mandibular primary molars. Ankylosis may also occur in the primary molars when there is no permanent successor. The child with ankylosis should be seen frequently; treatment will be described in Chapter 7.

ECTOPIC ERUPTION

Ectopic eruption of permanent teeth may result from trauma, infection of the primary teeth or irregular resorption of roots of the primary teeth. Infected primary incisors, if retained, will often cause the premature eruption of a permanent incisor into an abnormal position (Fig. 5–15). It has been shown by Kim, Shiere and Fogels that infected primary molars are responsible for malpositions and rotations of the premolars.

The most common site of irregular resorption of the roots of the primary molars is the distobuccal root of the maxillary primary second molar. This condition may also occur on the distal root of the mandibular

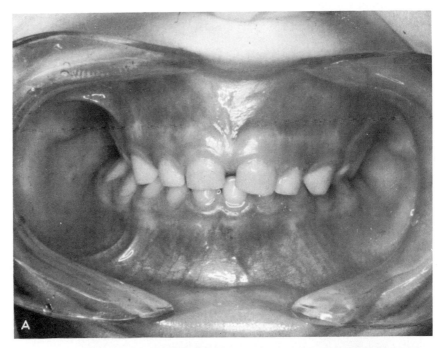

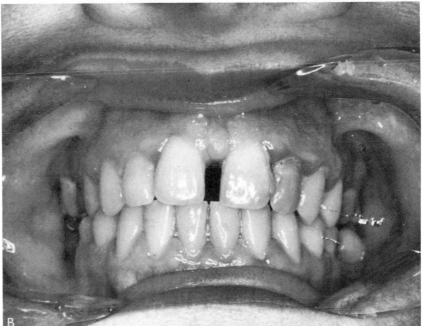

Figure 5–13

A, Four year old child with diastema between maxillary central incisors.
B, Patient's mother, showing a diastema between permanent central incisors.

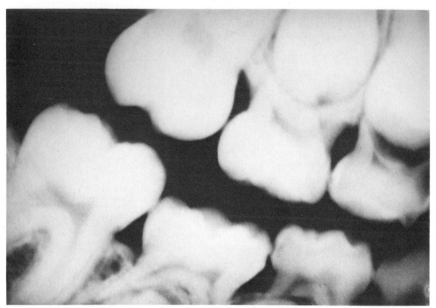

Figure 5–14. Ankylosis of mandibular first and second primary molars. Note discrepancy of occlusal plane of primary molars in relationship to first permanent molars.

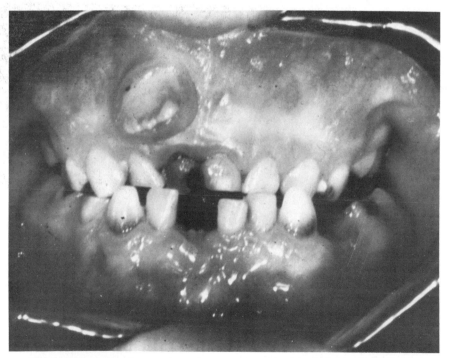

Figure 5–15. Ectopic eruption of permanent central incisors owing to traumatic injury of primary central incisors.

second primary molar. It may be seen as early as age 3 to 3½, and contributes to ectopic eruption of the first permanent molar. In ectopic eruption, the child should be seen frequently, but treatment is deferred until the first permanent molar has emerged. (See Chap. 7).

TREATMENT OF CLASS I DEEP OVERBITE IN THE PRIMARY DENTITION

Deep overbite in the primary dentition occurs frequently. Baume (1950), in his excellent report on the biogenic course of the primary dentition, stated that "there was no increase in interdental spacing in arches with spaced teeth and spacing never developed in which teeth are in contact." This has been my observation regarding spacing. Class I cases with deep overbite should be treated, since closed bite may interfere with the development of the intermaxillary space by retarding the ramus length growth.

It has been shown by Matthew (1959) that maxillary bite plates may be used for cases of deep overbite of the primary dentition when there is no spacing of the mandibular incisors. As well as having created spacing between these incisors he found that the intermaxillary space had increased and there was a marked improvement in occlusal relationships of the maxillary incisors to the mandibular incisors (Fig. 5–16).

The maxillary bite plate is highly recommended for closed bite cases in the primary dentition and will contribute to a more satisfactory development of the mixed and permanent dentitions.

TREATMENT OF SEVERE CLASS II OCCLUSAL DISHARMONIES IN THE PRIMARY DENTITION

True Class II occlusal disharmonies of the primary dentition should be treated with the understanding that this is only the first part of the treatment and that further treatment will be necessary in the mixed dentition.

When a patient with a Class II relationship presents with a protrusion of the maxillary arch and difficulty closing the lip over the maxillary primary incisors, severe overjet and overbite, and with the primary second mandibular molars are half a tooth or more distal to the maxillary second molars, treatment is highly recommended. Treatment will improve appearance, foster anteroposterior growth and allow both ramus length and satisfactory development of the intermaxillary space. Treatment of true Class II occlusal disharmonies of the primary dentition reduces and simplifies treatment of the mixed and early permanent dentition. Reports have stated that in some cases the distal movement of the primary molars may contribute to impaction of the maxillary first permanent molars. During treatment, if care is taken to keep the second primary molars upright and to move them distally in an upright position, the chances for impaction of the first permanent molars are negligible.

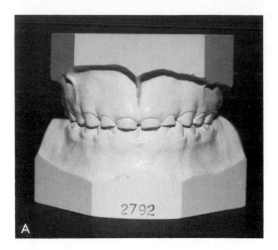

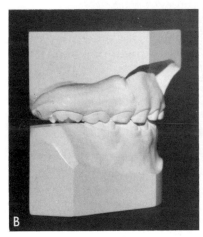
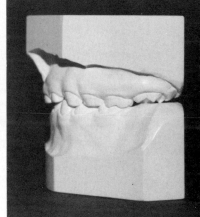

Figure 5–16

A, Casts of 5½ year old patient with deep overbite.
B, Lateral views.

Severe Class II occlusal disharmonies in the primary dentition respond favorably to treatment with cervical headgear appliance or banding of the maxillary incisors (Fig. 5–17).

In true Class II occlusal disharmonies there are varying degrees of overjet and overbite, and the child may have difficulty closing the lips without straining the lips over the maxillary incisors. There may be an adequate or inadequate arch length discrepancy.

In the cases in which there is adequate arch length, treatment may be accomplished in six months or longer. There is relatively little or no problem with arch length. All of these cases require further treatment, and the optimal time for treatment is when the permanent second molars begin to erupt.

If the arch length is inadequate, as seen in Figure 5–17, treatment is indicated. In this patient, when the permanent maxillary incisors erupted the arch length discrepancy became accentuated. The molar relationship remained in its corrected position until the patient reached the age of 8 years. Primary canines were then extracted and the permanent maxillary and mandibular incisors were aligned. Serial extractions were then car-

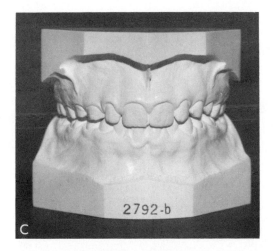

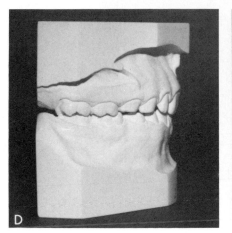
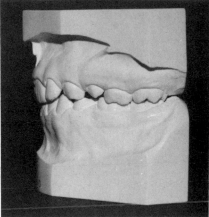

Figure 5–16 *Continued. C,* Casts of same patient approximately 1½ years later, after having worn a bite plate.

D, Note improvement of closed bite and development of the intermaxillary space.

(Courtesy of Dr. J. Rodney Mathews, Berkeley, California.)

ried out, and retreatment of the occlusal disharmony with multiband therapy resulted in a satisfactory occlusal relationship.

The treatment of Class II occlusal disharmonies in the primary dentition establishes an early satisfactory molar relationship which in the majority of cases remains stable. In those cases in which there are growth discrepancies treatment may be resumed before eruption of the second permanent molars to maintain a satisfactory molar relationship.

The retruded position of primary maxillary incisors provides a more suitable environment for the emergence and eruption of the permanent maxillary incisors.

Early treatment of Class II occlusal disharmonies has a beneficial effect on growth and development of the dentofacial complex once satisfactory anteroposterior occlusal relationship is established. Secondary treatment in Class II occlusal disharmonies invariably is indicated and usually is not difficult. The treatment in the mixed early permanent dentition is reduced and a more stable occlusal relationship of the permanent dentition may be anticipated.

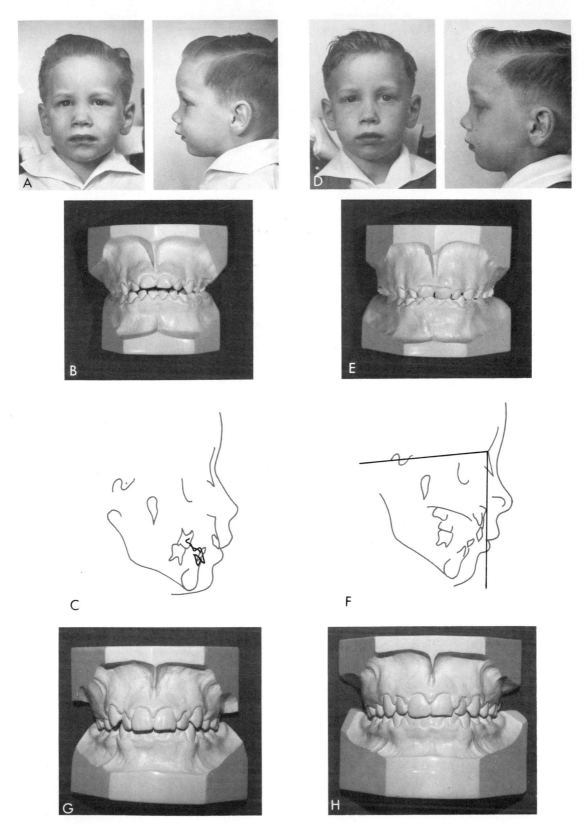

Figure 5-17

MAINTAINING ARCH LENGTH

It is most important to maintain arch length, particularly in the primary molars, which act as directional guideposts for the permanent premolars. When rampant caries are found in a child, one of the most effective ways of maintaining arch length is the fabrication of stainless steel crowns. Good operative procedures which maintain proximal contacts are most essential for the preservation of arch length.

Often, primary molars in younger children (ages 5 to 7 years) are pulpotomized or devitalized and remain asymptomatic. These teeth should be checked carefully radiographically. If they develop infections in the bifurcation or apical areas they should be extracted, since it has been shown by Kim, Shiere and Fogels that retained infected primary mandibular molars often contribute to rotations and divergencies in axial inclinations of the unerupted premolars. Infected primary mandibular molars or root fragments should never be allowed to remain in the mouth for the maintenance of arch length. When infected primary molars or root fragments are extracted, arch length may be maintained with either a fixed or a removable appliance.

OVERRETAINED PRIMARY INCISORS

If there is atypical resorption of the roots of the primary incisors, frequently the permanent central incisors will erupt lingually in the mandible and labially or lingually in the maxilla. This condition occurs more frequently in the mandible than in the maxilla. Extraction of these primary incisors will, in most instances, show resorption of the lingual aspect of the root. The labial root remnant prevents the primary incisor from being exfoliated. The overretained primary incisors should be extracted. If the permanent central incisors appear to be large it is wise to remove the four primary incisors. No further treatment is necessary since the pressure of the tongue will move the permanent incisors into the arch curve.

Figure 5–17

A, Photograph before treatment of a 4 year old boy with a severe Class II occlusal disharmony, showing difficulty in closing lips when in centric relationship.

B, Casts of same patient showing severe Class II relationship in primary dentition.

C, A cephalometric roentgenogram showing marked distal relationship of primary molars and protrusion of maxillary incisors with open bite.

D, Facial appearance of patient after treatment with headgear and multiband therapy. Note improvement and evidence of strain removed from the lips.

E, Casts of patient in centric occlusion after approximately 6 months of treatment with headgear and multiband therapy.

F, Cephalometric roentgenogram showing satisfactory molar relationship after treatment. Note improvement of facial profile and the retraction of the primary central incisors.

G, Casts of patient after serial extraction and alignment of permanent maxillary and mandibular incisors.

H, Casts of patient after treatment with multiband therapy.

(Courtesy of Dr. Eugene West, San Francisco, California.)

See illustration on opposite page.

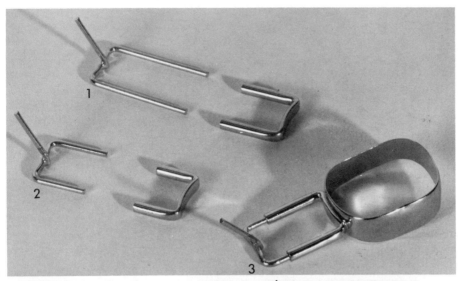

A

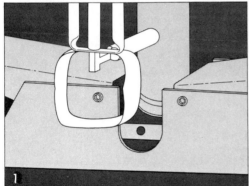

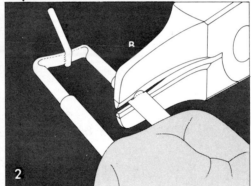

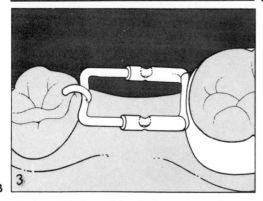

B

Figure 5–18

A, Different lengths of wires, tubes and lug rests *(1, 2)* before they are assembled and crimped or soldered to the *band* or *crown. 3,* Prewelded tube and band.

B, Fitting the direct space maintainer. *1,* Select a size and trial fit and mark the location on the mesial surface where the maintainer tube is to be attached. Remove crown or band and weld or solder the tube to the mesial surface. *2,* Insert maintainer wires into tube ends and trial fit the assembly. Crimp lightly to hold position. *3,* Remove assembly and crimp tubes firmly over the wires. A strong crimp on both sides will hold the wire securely. If desired, the junction may also be welded or soldered. Cement complete assembly and adapt, fitting as close to the edentulous space as possible to minimize occlusal forces on the maintainer. If an occlusal rest is used, bend it to the marginal ridge. If indicated, a small occlusal rest may be ground into the marginal ridge before fitting.

(Courtesy of Unitek Corporation.)

PREMATURE LOSS OF PRIMARY TEETH FROM CARIES OR TRAUMA

LOSS OF PRIMARY FIRST MOLARS

When primary first molars are lost prematurely it is essential to place the child under observation. In some instances there is no mesial drift to the primary second molars, whereas in other instances there is. Measurement of the space may be made with fine calipers and recorded on the child's chart at six month intervals. If in six months there is a mesial drift of 1 mm. or more, a space maintainer should be placed, utilizing the second primary molar. A very stable type of appliance is a crown and crib space maintainer. This crib is made with two arms, one on the buccal side and one on the lingual side abutting the primary canine. A direct space maintainer may be used as shown in Figure 5–18.

LOSS OF PRIMARY SECOND MOLARS

The premature loss of primary second molars creates a serious orthodontic problem, since there is mesial drifting of the first permanent

Figure 5–19

A, Different lengths of wires with distal shoes and tubes *(1, 2)* before they are assembled, crimped or soldered to band or crown. *3,* Prewelded tube and band.

B, Fitting maintainers with distal shoes when second primary molars are lost prematurely. After selecting the correct size first primary crown and preparing the tooth, insert distal shoe and trial fit the assembly. As with the standard maintainer, additional strength can be gained by using solder around the welded joint. Ideally, the tube assembly should be positioned on the crown at a level that allows the tooth in the opposing arch to just barely make contact, low enough to avoid subjecting the maintainer to excessive occlusal forces. If adapting to a healed edentulous space, the incision may be made with a sterile scalpel or other suitable instrument after examining the x-ray for proper position. When adapting after extraction, the maintainer is trial fitted, with the distal shoe in place, down the distal wall of the extraction socket. Prior to cementation, x-ray the appliance in the mouth. Make any necessary adjustments, then crimp both sides of the tube assembly to prevent further movement. Cement the appliance in place.

(Courtesy of Unitek Corporation.)

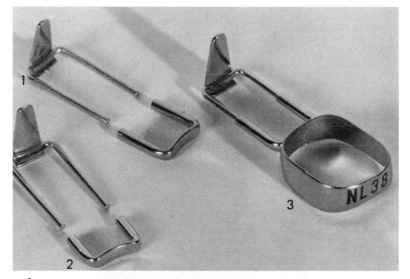

A

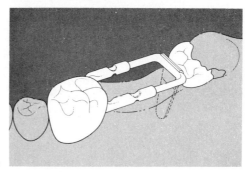

B

molars. This invariably creates an arch length loss, impacting the second permanent premolar. A stainless steel crown on the first premolar, and in some instances on the primary canine, with a horizontal bar and a cantilever arm may be constructed in a vertical plane to penetrate the gingiva mesial to the first permanent molar. A simple appliance is the Unitek space maintainer with the distal shoe (Figs. 5–19 and 5–20).

PROSTHESIS IN THE PRIMARY DENTITION

In children who have tooth agenesis, or in whom teeth are lost prematurely owing to dental caries or trauma, a full denture or a partial plastic denture, utilizing primary teeth may be made for the child and may serve well both esthetically and functionally (Cohen et al., in press) (Fig. 5–21). Children who lose their anterior teeth prematurely should have a temporary prosthesis fabricated, since they are sensitive about being "different" from other young children (Fig. 5–22). With the normal exfoliation of teeth, older children do not have this problem since their contemporaries are also shedding their primary teeth.

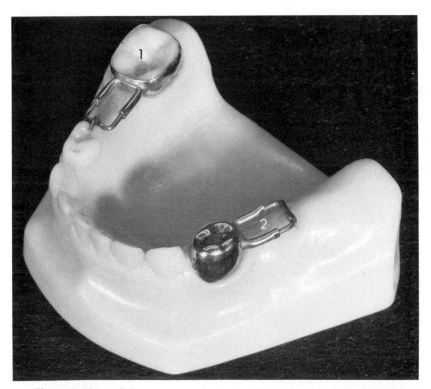

Figure 5–20. *1*. Direct space maintainer utilizing band cemented in place. *2*, Immediate space maintainer with distal shoe utilizing crown cemented into place.

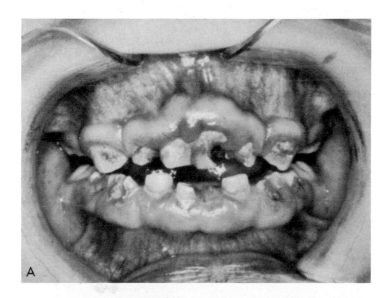

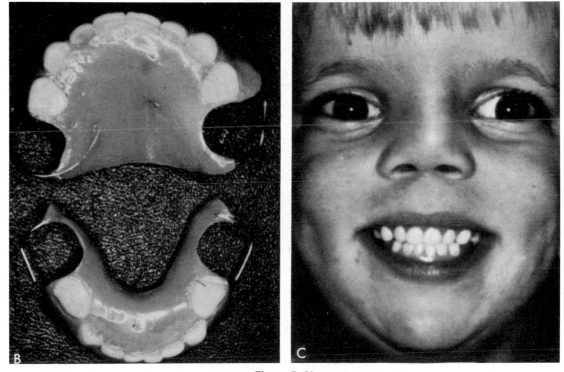

Figure 5–21

A, A 5¹/₂ year old Causasian male with fetal face syndrome, with numerous severely infected maxillary and mandibular primary teeth. Numerous teeth were extracted and crowns were placed on maxillary and mandibular second molars.

B, Partial dentures with wrought clasps.

C, Patient with dentures in occlusion.

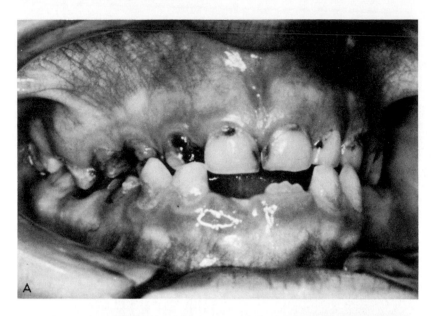

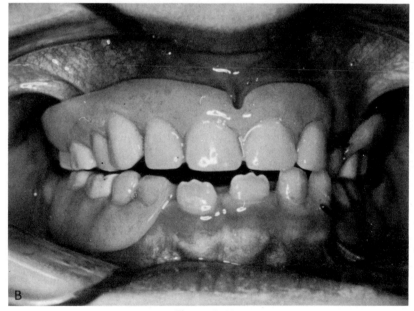

Figure 5–22

    A, A 6½ year old Caucasian male with numerous infected carious teeth, before treatment.

    B, Patient 6 months later, after infected teeth were removed and partial dentures inserted.

REFERENCES

Growth and Development

Baume, L. J.: Physiological tooth migration and its significance for the development of occlusion. J. Dent. Res., *29*:123–132, 1950.

Baume, L. J.: Developmental and diagnostic aspects of the primary dentition. Int. Dent. J., *9*:349–366, 1959.

Chapman, H.: The normal dental arch and its changes from birth to adult. Brit. Dent. J., *58*:201–209, 1951.

Clinch, L. M.: Serial models of two cases of normal occlusion between birth and four years. Dent. Res., *60*:323, 1940.

Clinch, L. M.: An analysis of serial models between three and eight years of age. Dent. Res., *71*:61–72, 1951.
Clinch, L. M.: Early treatment of a prenormal mandible. Dent. Pract., *14*, 1963.
Clinch, L. M., et al.: Symposium on aspects of the dental development of the child. Dent. Pract., *17*, 1966.
Cohen, J. T.: Growth and development of the dental arches in children. J.A.D.A., *27*:1250, 1940.
Cohen, M. M., Jr., Needleman, H. L., and Cohen, M. M., Sr.: The fetal face syndrome. J. Med. Genet. (in press).
Coughlin, J. W.: Sex differences in the prenatal human deciduous molar crown. J. Dent. Res., *46*:554–558, 1967.
Coyler, F.: A note on the changes in the dental arch during childhood. Dent. Record, *40*:273–281, 1920.
Foster, T. D., and Hamilton, M. D.: Occlusion in the primary dentition: Study of children 2½ to 3 years of age. Brit. Dent. J., *126*:76–79, 1968.
Foster, T. D., Hamilton, M. D. and La Velle, C. L. B.: Dentition and dental arch dimension in British children at the age of 2½ and 3 years. Arch. Oral Biol., *14*:1031–1040, 1969.
Freil, S.: The development of ideal occlusion of the gum pads and the teeth. Am. J. Orthod., *40*:196–227, 1954.
Holcomb, A. E., and Meredith, H. V.: Width of the dental arches at the deciduous canines in white children 4 to 8 years of age. Growth, *20*:159–177, 1966.
Humphrey, H. F., and Leighton, B. C.: Survey of anteroposterior abnormalities of the jaws in children between the ages of 2 and 5½ years of age. Brit. Dent. J., *88*:3, 1950.
Jorgenson, K. D.: The deciduous dentition: A descriptive and anatomical study. Acta. Odont. Scand., *14*: Suppl. 20, 1956.
Kim, T. H., Shiere, F. R., and Fogels, H. R.: Pre-eruptive factors of tooth rotation and axial inclination. J. Dent. Res., *40*:548–557, 1961.
Korhaus, G.: Clinical studies on the odontogenic development of the dentition. Dent. Record, *58*:641, 1938.
Massler, M., and Schour, I.: Studies in tooth development: Theories of eruption. Am. J. Orthod., *27*:552, 1941.
Matthew, J. R.: Malocclusion in the primary dentition. Dent. Clin. N. Amer., pp. 463, 478, July, 1966.
Meredith, H. V., and Hupp, W. M.: A longitudinal study of dental arch width at the deciduous second molars on children 4 to 8 years of age. J. Dent. Res., *35*:879–889, 1956.
Moorrees, C. F. A., Thomsen, S. Ø., Jensen, E., and Yen, P. K. J.: Mesiodistal crown diameters of the deciduous and permanent teeth in individuals. J. Dent. Res., *36*:39–47, 1957.
Nanda, R. S., Khan, I., and Anand, R.: Age changes in the occlusal pattern of deciduous dentition. J. Dent. Res., *52*:221–224, 1973.
Sanin, C., Blim, S. S., Clarkson, Q. C., and Thomas, D. R.: Prediction of occlusion by measurements of the deciduous dentition. Am. J. Orthod., *57*:561–572, 1970.
Sillman, J. H.: Serial study of occlusion. Am. J. Orthod., *34*:969, 1948.
Sillman, J H.: Serial study of good occlusion from birth to 12 years of age. Am. J. Orthod., *37*:7, 481, 1950.
Cohen, M. M., Shapiro, E., and Green, L. B.: Distribution of malocclusion in 443 preschool children in Brookline, Massachusetts. Unpublished data, 1953.
Foster, T. D., and Hamilton, M. C.: Occlusion in the primary dentition. Brit. Dent. J., *126*:76–79, 1969.
Haryett, R. D.: Malocclusion in public health. J. Canad. Dent., *28*:372–386, 1962.

Anomalies

Brook, A. H., and Winter, G. B.: Double teeth—a retrospective study of "geminated" and "fused" teeth in children. Brit. Dent. J., *129*:123–130, 1970.
Daush-Neumann, D.: Diastema with missing deciduous incisors. Fortsche Kieferorthop., *30*:82–88, 1969.
Gysel, C.: Mesiodentes familiaes. Rev. Belg. Med. Dent., *18*:929–960, 1963.
Gysel, C.: Mesiodentes temporares. Rev. Franç. Odontomat., *10*:957–969, 1963.
Hüsgen, W.: Zur Klink und kieferorthopädichen Behandlung der durch sogennte Mesiodentes verursachten Entwicklungsstörungen im Gebiet der oberen Frontzähne, Internes Festheft zum, 65, Geburtstag, Prov. Meyers, Göttingen, 1961 (unpublished).
Lind, V.: Mefödda antalsvariationer i permamenta dentitionen. Odont. Rev. (Malmo) 10:176–189, 1959.
Menczer, L. F.: Anomalies of the primary dentition. J. Dent., *22*:57–62, 1955.
Rune, B.: Submerged deciduous molars. Odont. Rev. (Malmo), *22*:257–73, 1971.
Weber, F.: Supernumerary teeth. Dent. Clin. N. Am., pp. 509–517, July, 1964.

Ankylosis

Aisenberg, M. S.: Studies of retained deciduous teeth. Am. J. Orthod., *27*:179, 1941.
Biederman, W.: Ankylosis. Ann. Dent. *12*:1–15, 1953.

Biederman, W.: The incidence and etiology of teeth ankylosis. Am. J. Orthod., *42*:921, 1956.

Biederman, W.: The problem of the ankylosed tooth. Dent. Clin. N. Am., pp. 409–424, July, 1968.

Brearley, L. J., and McKibben, D. H.: Ankylosis of primary molar teeth. I. Prevalence and Characteristics. II. A longitudinal study. J. Dent. Child. *40*:54–63, 1973.

Darling, A. I., and Levers, B. G.: Submerged human deciduous molars and ankylosis. Arch. Oral Biol., *18*:1021–1040, 1973.

Noyes, F. E.: Submerging deciduous molars. Angle Orthod., *2*:77–87, 1932.

Parker, W. S., Frisbe, H. E., and Grant, T. S.: The experimental production of dental ankylosis. Angle Orthod., *34*:103, 1964.

Rule, J. T., Zacherl, W. A., and Pfefferle, A. M.: The relationship between ankylosed molars and multiple enamel defects. J. Dent. Child., *39*:29–35, 1972.

Rygh, P., and Reitan, K.: Changes in the supporting tissues of submerged deciduous molars with and without permanent successors. Odont. Tskr., *72*:345, 1964.

Sharway, A. M., Mills, P. B., and Gibbons, R.: Multiple ankylosis occurring in rat teeth. Oral Surg., *26*:896, 1968.

Shaw, J., and Samuels, H. S.: The "submerged" tooth. Oral Surg., *14*:440–441, 1961.

Thornton, M., and Zimmerman, E. R.: Ankylosis of primary teeth. J. Dent. Child., *31*:120–126, 1964.

Via, W. F.: Submerged deciduous molars: Familial tendencies. J.A.D.A., *69*:127–129, 1964.

Vorhies, J., Gregory, T., and McDonald, R. E.: Ankylosed deciduous molars. J.A.D.A., *44*:68–72, 1952.

Habits

Bell, D., and Hale, A.: Observations of tongue-thrust swallow in pre-school children. J. Speech Hear. Disord., *28*:195–197, 1963.

Calisti, L. N., Cohen, M. M., and Fales, M.: Correlation between malocclusion, oral habits and socio-economic level of pre-school children. J. Dent. Res., *39*:450–454, 1960.

Hanson, M. L., Barnard, L. W., and Case, J. L.: Tongue thrust in preschool children. Am. J. Orthod., *56*:60–69, 1969.

Hanson, M. L., Barnard, L. W., and Case, J. L.: Tongue thrust in preschool children. Part II. Dental occlusion patterns. Am. J. Orthod., *57*:15–22, 1970.

Hanson, M. L., Barnard, L. W., and Case, J. L.: Tongue thrust in preschool children. Part III. Cinefluorographic analysis. Am. J. Orthod., *58*:268–275, 1970.

Kapoor, D. N., Roy, R. K., and Bagghi, M. K.: Effects of deleterious oral habits on the dentofacial complex. Indian J. Pediat., *37*:102, 1970.

Lewis, J. A., and Counihan, R. F.: Tongue thrust in infancy. J. Speech Hear. Disord., *30*:280–282, 1965.

Moore, G. J., McNeill, R. W., and D'Anna, J. A.: The effects of digit sucking on facial growth. J.A.D.A., *84*:592–599, 1972.

Nanda, R. S., Khan, I., and Anand, R.: Effect of oral habits on the occlusion in pre-school children. J. Dent. Child., *39*:31–34, 1972.

Sillman, J. H.: Finger-sucking: serial dental study from birth to five years. N.Y. State J. Med., *42*:2024–2028, 1942.

Treatment

Breitner, C.: The influence of moving deciduous teeth on the permanent successors. Am. J. Orthod. Oral Surg., *26*:1152, 1940.

Hahn, G.: Treatment in the deciduous dentition. Am. J. Orthod., *41*:255, 1955.

Kelstein, L. B.: Correction of Class II malocclusion with open bite in the primary dentition. J. Dent. Child., *28*:89–91, 1961.

Matthew, J. R.: Maxillary bite plane application in Class I deciduous occlusion. Am. J. Orthod., *45*:721–737, 1959.

Matthew, J. R.: Translocational movement of first deciduous molars into second molar positions. Am. J. Orthod., *55*:276–285, 1969.

Rinderer, L.: Care of the deciduous teeth, orthodontic diagnosis and treatment expectations. Rev. Belg. Med. Dent., *24*:123–128, 1969.

Watson, D. H.: Orthodontics and the growing child—problems encountered in the primary dentition. Int. J. Orthod., *7*:68–75, 1969.

Waugh, L. M.: Care of the deciduous teeth as the basis of occlusion of the permanent dentition. Am. J. Orthod., *41*:90–106, 1955.

West, E. E.: Treatment objectives in the deciduous dentition. Am. J. Orthod., *55*:617–632, 1969.

6

Recognition, Diagnosis and Treatment of Class II Occlusal Disharmonies

JOHN ORR

This chapter will deal with the recognition and diagnosis of Class II disharmonies in the mixed dentition. Children with a Class II molar occlusion, complicated by protruding incisors, are more prone to suffer fractures of the anterior teeth. The prevention of fractured teeth, as well as the interception of an occlusal and facial disharmony, makes the recognition and early treatment of Class II problems mandatory. It is the aim of mixed dentition treatment to guide the teeth during eruption so that the dentition may develop to its maximum dimensions and result in a harmonious occlusion. The optimum time to treat certain Class II occlusal disharmonies is in the early mixed dentition in children between the ages of 7 and 9 years. Before treating Class II occlusal disharmonies in the mixed dentition the dentist must determine whether the lower arch is an accommodating arch, and if there will be space for the succedaneous teeth to erupt without crowding or protruding lower incisors.

DIAGNOSIS

In analytical diagnosis of the mixed dentition, the arch perimeter must be carefully evaluated. Additional perimeter for the larger permanent incisors is gained when the following factors are present:

1. Space between the primary incisors.
2. Intercanine growth by apposition of bone on the lateral aspects of the alveolus.
3. Labial inclination of permanent incisors.

It is most important for the dentist to understand the difference between a satisfactory occlusion for a particular stage of development and what may be considered an unsatisfactory occlusion. What may appear to be an occlusal disharmony might actually be normal for that particular stage of development. For example, there is often an end-to-end molar relationship in the mixed dentition, which some dentists may erroneously consider an incipient Class II occlusal disharmony. It is not until after the primary molars are lost that the final relationship of the permanent molars usually develops. This shifting of the molar occlusion from an apparent Class II tendency to a satisfactory Class I relationship is due to the "leeway space," as suggested by Nance (1947). Nance found that the combined width of the primary canine and primary molars averages 1.7 mm. more in the mandibular arch and 0.9 mm. more in the maxillary arch than the combined widths of their permanent successors measure. When primary maxillary and mandibular molars are lost prematurely it is sometimes necessary to preserve this leeway space. Failure to preserve this space frequently results in mesial migration of the first permanent molars. This may be prevented by the insertion of a maxillary and a mandibular passive lingual arch wire.

When a Class II occlusal relationship is observed in the primary dentition, study casts should be made, and the child should be placed under orthodontic observation. A true Class II relationship with or without an excessive overbite rarely corrects itself and invariably becomes accentuated after the eruption of the permanent incisors. A successful analytical diagnosis depends upon the evaluation of the mandibular arch, including a mixed dentition analysis and a cephalometric analysis.

EVALUATION OF THE MANDIBULAR ARCH

Available Space

The available space measurement is made by adapting a piece of soft 0.020 or 0.022 in. brass wire from the mesial surface of the right mandibular first molar to the mesial surface of the left mandibular first molar, forming it to lie over the buccal cusps of the primary molars and the incisal edges of the mandibular permanent incisors. The wire is then straightened and measured in millimeters and recorded as available space.

ILLUSTRATION OF MIXED DENTITION ANALYSIS

A mixed dentition analysis will provide information on whether there will be sufficient space for the unerupted canines and first and second premolars. Moyers and Jenkins' mixed dentition analysis has the following advantages:

1. The possibility of error is minimal, and the range of error may be calculated.
2. It is not time consuming.
3. It requires no special equipment.
4. It may be done on actual teeth or on casts.
5. It may be used for both arches.

The approximate size of the mandibular canines and premolars is calculated by measuring the erupted permanent incisor teeth. The combined mesiodistal diameter measurement of the mandibular incisors and the estimated size of the canines and premolars bilaterally constitutes the required space for the permanent dentition. This evaluation has a high degree of accuracy, since there is a close correlation between the mesiodistal dimension of the mandibular incisors and the mesiodistal diameters of the mandibular canines and premolars.

The total mesiodistal widths of the permanent incisors are measured

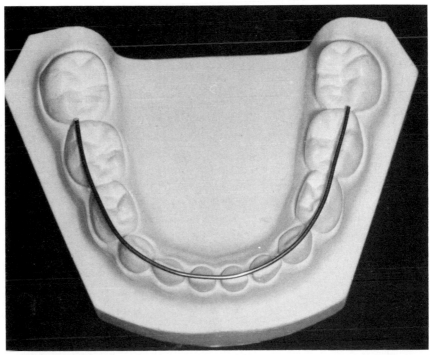

Figure 6–1. Soft 22 gauge brass wire is bent to lie over the tips of the incisor teeth and buccal cusps of the primary molars. The wire ends in the embrasure between second and primary molars and first permanent molar.

and the results are located on the probability chart designed by Moyers and Jenkins. The measurements on this chart begin at 19.5 mm. and continue to 29 mm., with 0.5 mm. gradations. Each measurement corresponds to a comparable percentile of estimated canine and premolar widths found in the general population. Following is an example of how the chart may be used. When the combined incisor width is 22.0 mm., 95 per cent of the population would have an approximate combined canine and premolar width of 22.6 mm. or less. When the canine and premolar widths total 21.6 mm. or less, only 75 per cent of the population would have a combined width of 22.6 mm. (Table 6–1).

TABLE 6–1. PROBABILITY CHART FOR PREDICTING THE SUM OF THE WIDTHS OF 345 FROM $\overline{21|12}$.*

∑21/12 =	19.5	20.0	20.5	21.0	21.5	22.0	22.5	23.0	23.5	24.0	24.5	25.0	25.5	26.0	26.5	27.0	27.5	28.0	28.5	29.0
95%	21.6	21.8	22.1	22.4	22.7	22.9	23.2	23.5	23.8	24.0	24.3	24.6	24.9	25.1	25.4	25.7	26.0	26.2	26.5	26.7
85%	21.0	21.3	21.5	21.8	22.1	22.4	22.6	22.9	23.2	23.5	23.7	24.0	24.3	24.6	24.8	25.1	25.4	25.7	25.9	26.2
75%	20.6	20.9	21.2	21.5	21.8	22.0	22.3	22.6	22.9	23.1	23.4	23.7	24.0	24.2	24.5	24.8	25.0	25.3	25.6	25.9
65%	20.4	20.6	20.9	21.2	21.5	21.8	22.0	22.3	22.6	22.8	23.1	23.4	23.7	24.0	24.2	24.5	24.8	25.1	25.3	25.6
50%	20.0	20.3	20.6	20.8	21.1	21.4	21.7	21.9	22.2	22.5	22.8	23.0	23.3	23.6	23.9	24.1	24.4	24.7	25.0	25.3
35%	19.6	19.9	20.2	20.5	20.8	21.0	21.3	21.6	21.9	22.1	22.4	22.7	23.0	23.2	23.5	23.8	24.1	24.3	24.6	24.9
25%	19.4	19.7	19.9	20.2	20.5	20.8	21.0	21.3	21.6	21.9	22.1	22.4	22.7	23.0	23.2	23.5	23.8	24.1	24.3	24.6
15%	19.0	19.3	19.6	19.9	20.2	20.7	21.0	21.3	21.5	21.8	22.1	22.1	22.6	22.9	23.2	23.4	23.7	24.0	24.3	
5%	18.5	18.8	19.0	19.3	19.6	19.9	20.1	20.4	20.7	21.0	21.2	21.5	21.8	22.1	22.3	22.6	22.9	23.2	23.4	23.7

PROBABILITY CHART FOR PREDICTING THE SUM OF THE WIDTHS OF $\overline{345}$ FROM $\overline{21/12}$

∑21/12 =	19.5	20.0	20.5	21.0	21.5	22.0	22.5	23.0	23.5	24.0	24.5	25.0	25.5	26.0	26.5	27.0	27.5	28.0	28.5	29.0
95%	21.1	21.4	21.7	22.0	22.3	22.6	22.9	23.2	23.5	23.8	24.1	24.4	24.7	25.0	25.3	25.6	25.8	26.1	26.4	26.7
85%	20.5	20.8	21.1	21.4	21.7	22.0	22.3	22.6	22.9	23.2	23.5	23.8	24.0	24.3	24.6	24.9	25.2	25.5	25.8	26.1
75%	20.1	20.4	20.7	21.0	21.3	21.6	21.9	22.2	22.5	22.8	23.1	23.4	23.7	24.0	24.3	24.6	24.8	25.1	25.4	25.7
65%	19.8	20.1	20.4	20.7	21.0	21.3	21.6	21.9	22.2	22.5	22.8	23.1	23.4	23.7	24.0	24.3	24.6	24.8	25.1	25.4
50%	19.4	19.7	20.0	20.3	20.6	20.9	21.2	21.5	21.8	22.1	22.4	22.7	23.0	23.3	23.6	23.9	24.2	24.5	24.7	25.0
35%	19.0	19.3	19.6	19.9	20.2	20.5	20.8	21.1	21.4	21.7	22.0	22.3	22.6	22.9	23.2	23.5	23.8	24.0	24.3	24.6
25%	18.7	19.0	19.3	19.6	19.9	20.2	20.5	20.8	21.1	21.4	21.7	22.0	22.3	22.6	22.9	23.2	23.5	23.8	24.1	24.4
15%	18.4	18.7	19.0	19.3	19.6	19.8	20.1	20.4	20.7	21.0	21.3	21.6	21.9	22.2	22.5	22.8	23.1	23.4	23.7	24.0
5%	17.7	18.0	18.3	18.6	18.9	19.2	19.5	19.8	20.1	20.4	20.7	21.0	21.3	21.6	21.9	22.2	22.5	22.8	23.1	23.4

*From Moyers, 1963.

Recently Watson (1972) has suggested a formula for a rapid and more accurate assessment of the mesiodistal diameters of unerupted canines and premolars. A standard algebraic proportion system is used for this evaluation. It is necessary to take a measurement of a primary tooth on the study cast and a measurement from a radiograph of both the unerupted tooth and the same erupted tooth that is measured on the cast. The radiographic measurements of the erupted tooth must be taken from the same radiograph as that of the unerupted tooth. The following are examples of the algebraic proportions system for determining mesiodistal diameters of unerupted teeth.

$$\frac{U_1}{U_2} = \frac{E_1}{E_2}$$

Where U_1 = actual width of unerupted tooth
U_2 = width of unerupted tooth (measured on radiograph)
E_1 = width of erupted primary tooth (measured on study cast)
E_2 = width of erupted primary tooth (measured on same radiograph)

For example, the proportion for determining the M-D width of the mandibular second premolar would be:

$$\frac{\text{M-D width of } \underline{5}\ (X)}{\text{M-D width of } \underline{5} \text{ (on the radiograph)}} = \frac{\text{M-D width of primary second molar (on study cast)}}{\text{M-D width of primary second molar (on the same radiograph)}}$$

We insert the values called for by the proportion:

$$\frac{X}{8.5 \text{ mm. (from radiograph)}} = \frac{9.4 \text{ mm. (from study cast)}}{10.0 \text{ mm. (from same radiograph)}}$$

Next we cross multiply:

$$10X = 8.5 \times 9.4$$
$$10X = 79.90 \text{ or}$$
$$X = 7.99 \text{ mm. (M-D width of } \underline{5})$$

The proportion can be used for any unerupted tooth in the dental arch, upper as well as lower. All that must be done is to insert the proper figures in the proportion and cross multiply. It is mandatory that the two radiographic measurements be taken from the same radiograph. If it is necessary to determine the width of a canine, the proportion could be modified to read:

$$\frac{\text{M-D width of } \underline{3}\ (X)}{\text{M-D width of } \underline{3} \text{ (on radiograph)}} = \frac{\text{M-D width of } \underline{2} \text{ (on study cast)}}{\text{M-D width of } \underline{2} \text{ (on same radiograph)}}$$

To find the width of an upper lateral tooth we can use this proportion:

$$\frac{\text{M-D width of } \underline{2}\ (X)}{\text{M-D width of } \underline{2} \text{ (on radiograph)}} = \frac{\text{M-D width of } \underline{II} \text{ *(on study cast)}}{\text{M-D width of } \underline{2} \text{ (on same radiograph)}}$$

The x-ray distortion factor is no longer a problem since it appears on both sides of the proportion and cancels itself out.

A comparison is now made between the *required* space and the *available* space. When the required space is equal or slightly less than the available space, minimal treatment may be anticipated since there is sufficient room for the permanent molars to move mesially and for the permanent canines and premolars to erupt into the dental arch without crowding.

---

*Primary tooth (lateral).

CEPHALOMETRIC ANALYSIS

Another factor which must be considered in the evaluation of available space is the position of the mandibular incisors.

Williams (1969) has suggested a simple method for evaluating the labiolingual position of the mandibular incisors utilizing a cephalometric roentgenogram. One cephalometric criterion common to a harmonious, well-balanced profile in the majority of individuals is the relationship of the mandibular incisor to the anteroposterior (AP) line (Figs. 6–2, 6–3, and 6–4).

In the cephalometric analysis the tip of the lower incisor is drawn on the tracing paper, and the distance in millimeters to the AP line is measured. The incisor tip may fall on, in front of or behind the AP line. If the incisor tip lies anterior to the AP line, and the required space is equal to or greater than the available space, this patient probably would not be a candidate for headgear treatment. The indications are that reduction of tooth material may be necessary later in order to have a harmonious facial profile. If the position of the lower incisor tip is posterior to the AP line, the arch length may be increased by moving the lower incisors out to the line. For every millimeter of anterior tooth movement 2 mm. in arch length is gained. This type of Class II occlusal disharmony may often be treated successfully without premolar extraction with the use of headgear therapy, which effectively corrects the Class II molar relationship and protruding maxillary incisors.

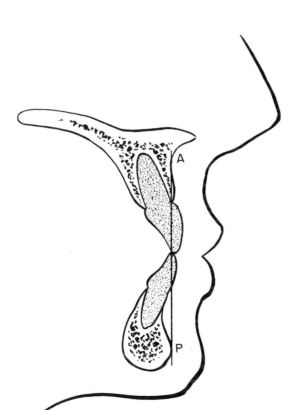

Figure 6–2. This drawing shows a satisfactory position of the tip of the lower incisor on the AP line.

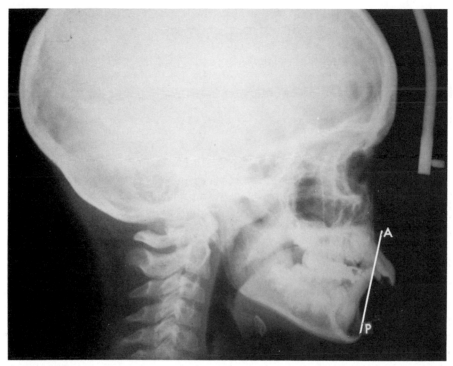

Figure 6–3. A satisfactory cephalometric profile in the mixed dentition of a patient with a Class II division I occlusal disharmony. Headgear treatment may be considered since the tips of the mandibular incisors are behind or distal to the AP line before treatment.

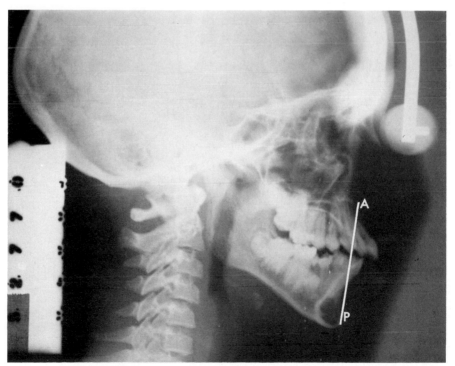

Figure 6–4. A cephalometric roentgenogram of a mixed dentition showing mandibular incisors that lie in front of or mesial to the AP line before treatment. This type of occlusal disharmony should not be considered for headgear therapy in the mixed dentition since it may result in a bimaxillary protrusion.

The evaluation of the mandibular arch and cephalometric analysis are only guides for the practitioner in determining the need for early treatment of Class II occlusal disharmonies.

In a recent seminar on management of moderate occlusal disharmonies Swain (1971) suggested the following guidelines for headgear treatment in the mixed dentition for Class II division 1 occlusal disharmony:

1. Broad dental arches.
2. No tooth-to-jaw discrepancy in lower arch.
3. Flat lower occlusal plane or shallow curve.
4. Lower incisor within −1 mm. to +2 mm. in relation to the AP line.
5. Lower anteriors upright and in good alignment.
6. Alternatively, lower teeth may be aligned, except that the anteriors have mild lingual inclinations combined with slight irregularity.
7. Patient is willing to wear headgear at least 23 hours a day.

Swain believes that favorable results depend upon the forward and downward growth of the dentofacial complex and on the constant restraint on the maxilla by the headgear.

The before-and-after models in Figures 6–5 and 6–9 show children with developing Class II problems that were intercepted in the mixed dentition and treated using extraoral anchorage as the principal appliance. All of these patients also had the maxillary incisors banded, a twin wire type arch placed and Class II elastics to the mandibular lingual arch wire.

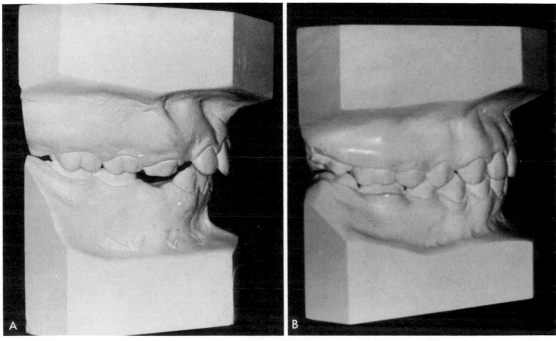

Figure 6–5

A, Casts of patient showing Class II molar relationship and closed bite before treatment.

B, Case after treatment with headgear therapy, a twin wire arch on the maxillary incisors, and a mandibular anchorage lingual arch wire. Class II elastics were worn when headgear was not in place.

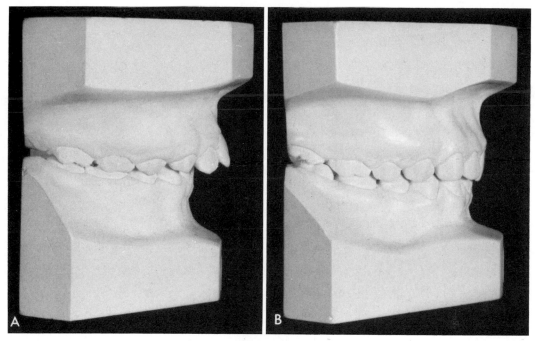

Figure 6–6

A, The maxillary casts before treatment showed a severe protrusion of the maxillary anterior teeth and a closed bite, Class II molar and canine relationships.

B, Casts after treatment. Note reduction of the protrusion and bite opening. Treatment consisted of headgear, twin wire type arch on maxillary teeth, and a mandibular anchorage lingual arch. Treatment time was 16 months.

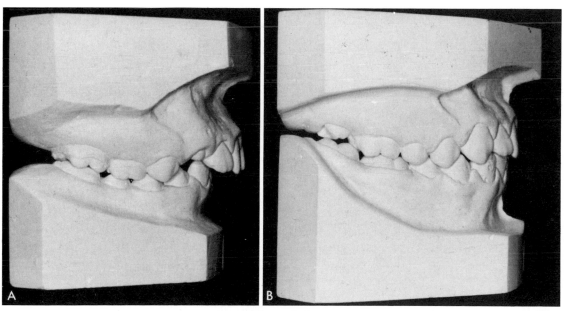

Figure 6–7

A, In this case note that the mandibular primary molar had been lost and the maxillary primary molar was retained. When the maxillary second molar is lost the permanent maxillary first molar will move into more mesial position than is observed on the cast of this case. This occlusal disharmony has protruding maxillary incisors, closed bite, and a canine position observed in Class II division I occlusal disharmony.

B, Casts after treatment with twin wire type arch on maxillary incisors, headgear, and mandibular anchorage lingual arch utilizing Class II elastics. Treatment time was 18 months.

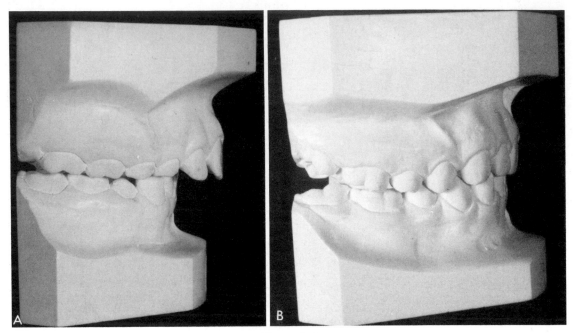

Figure 6–8

A, Casts of Class II division I occlusal disharmony before treatment. Note closed bite and maxillary protrusion.

B, Treatment included headgear therapy, sliding Class II hook on a maxillary twin wire arch, mandibular lingual anchorage arch, and mandibular twin wire arch. Note the satisfactory occlusal relationship and the opening of the bite when treatment was completed.

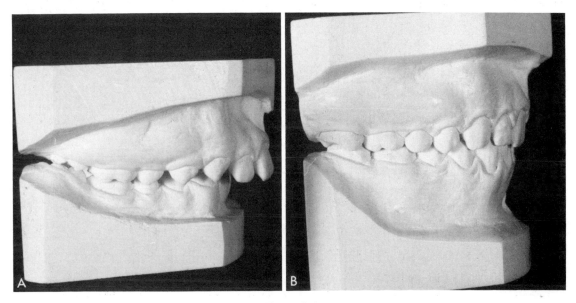

Figure 6–9

A, Cast of patient before treatment—Class II division I occlusal disharmony.

B, Cast of patient after treatment. Although treatment of this patient was started in the early adult dentition, complete reduction of the protrusion and opening of the bite was obtained without extractions. Only headgear therapy and Johnson type maxillary twin arch were used for completion of this case.

SUMMARY

The decision to treat Class II disharmonies in the mixed dentition depends on the evaluation of the mandibular arch. This evaluation can be accomplished by determining the available space, as suggested by Nance, and the required space, employing either the mixed dentition analysis M.D.A.) of Moyers and Jenkins or the standard algebraic proportion system (S.A.P.S.) suggested by Watson.

To make the M.D.A. more accurate, it must be corrected by doing a cephalometric analysis to determine the position of the lower incisor teeth in a labiolingual direction.

REFERENCES

Buchin, I. D.: Facial esthetics and cephalometric criteria as the determinant in the extraction decision. J. Clin. Orthod., 5:377–378; 385–393; 421–434; 481–491, 1971.

Burstone, D. J.: Distinguishing developing malocclusion from normal occlusion. Dent. Clin. N. Am., pp. 479–491, July, 1964.

Dewel, B. F.: The clinical application of the edgewise appliance in orthodontic treatment. Am. J. Orthod., 42:4–28, 1956.

Dewey, M.: Anchorage and Attachment. Int. J. Orthod., Oral Surg., 5:693, 1919.

Drenker, E. W.: Unilateral cervical traction with a Kloehn extraoral mechanism. Angle Orthod., 29:201–205, 1959.

Graber, T. M.: Upper second molar extraction in orthodontics treatment. Am. J. Orthod., 41:354–361, 1955.

Huckaba, G. W.: Arch size analysis and tooth size prediction. Dent. Clin. N. Am., pp. 431–440, July, 1964.

Kloehn, S. J.: Mixed dentition treatment. Angle Orthod., 20:75–96, 1950.

Kloehn, S. J.: At what age should treatment be started? Am. J. Orthod., 41:262–278, 1955.

Lewis, T. E.: Incidence of fractured anterior teeth as related to their protrusion. Angle Orthod., 29:131, 1959.

Mayne, W. R.: A concept, a diagnosis and a discipline. Dent. Clin. N. Am., pp. 281–288, July, 1959.

Mershon, J. V.: Physiology and mechanics in orthodontia. Dent. Cosmos, 10:1197, 1922.

Moorrees, C. F.A., and Chadha, J. M.: Available space for the incisors during dental development. A growth study based on physiological age. Angle Orthod., 35:12–22, 1965.

Mosmann, W. H.: Diagnosis and treatment with occipital anchorage. Am. J. Orthod., 42:112–115, 1956.

Moyers, R. E.: Handbook of Orthodontics. 2nd Ed. Chicago, Year Book Medical Publishers, 1963.

Nance, H. N.: The limitations of orthodontic treatment. Part I. Am. J. Orthod., 33:177–223, 253–301, 1947.

Nelson, B.: What does extraoral anchorage accomplish? Am. J. Orthod., 38:422–434, 1952.

Renfroe, E. W.: The factor of stabilization in anchorage. Am. J. Orthod., 42:883–897, 1956.

Ricketts, R. M.: The influence of orthodontic treatment on facial growth and development. Angle Orthod., 30:103–133, 1960.

Swain, B. F.: Borderline extraction cases. Guidelines for early treatment, headgear, treatment, serial extractions without immediate treatment, nonextraction trial, and one arch extraction treatment. J. Clin. Orthod. 10:539–565, 1971.

Taylor, W. H., and Hitchcock, P. H.: The Alabama analysis. Am. J. Orthod., 52:265–345, 1966.

Watson, D. H.: A rapid and accurate assessment of the mesial-distal dimensions of any unerupted permanent tooth. Int. J. Orthod., 10:91–92, 1972.

Weber, F. N.: Some clinical applications of the modified Johnson twin arch wire technique. Am. J. Orthod., 43:90–102, 1957.

Williams, R.: The diagnostic line. Am. J. Orthod., 55:458–476, 1969.

7

Minor Tooth Movement in the Early and Mixed Permanent Dentitions

After the exfoliation of the primary incisors, and the emergence and eruption of the permanent incisors, the practitioner has an unusual opportunity to observe early discrepancies in the occlusion. In many instances he may treat deviations and in this way prevent severe occlusal disharmonies.

The majority of primary dentitions have satisfactory Class I occlusal relationships. When the primary incisors are exfoliated, often there will be irregularities of the permanent incisor eruption pattern. When there is a discrepancy between tooth size of the primary and permanent incisors, there will be a lack of space to accommodate the larger permanent incisors. Oral habits also can influence the position of the emerging and developing permanent incisors.

A small percentage of primary dentitions have Class II relationships, particularly when the second primary mandibular molars are half a tooth or more distal to the maxillary primary molars. This type of occlusion is not self-correcting and, as the dentition develops, the Class II occlusal disharmony becomes more pronounced. The optimal time to treat Class II occlusal disharmonies is in the early mixed dentition. Chapter 6 was devoted to the early recognition of Class II occlusal disharmonies in the mixed dentition, and a method of treatment was carefully described.

Serial extractions in Class II disharmonies are sometimes indicated and when there is insufficient arch length to accommodate the premolars or when the primary canines are lost prematurely and there is a mesial migration of the primary first molars in one or both arches. In many instances the permanent canines will erupt in a labial position outside the arch, with the first premolars advanced in the arch. When serial extractions are contemplated, it is foolhardy to expect that the removal of the permanent first premolars will result in a self-correction of labially disposed canines or that a simple Hawley with a finger spring will correct the malposed canine. In most cases in which serial extractions are indicated they require long-term observation followed by complete orthodontic treatment. This short summary of serial extractions will be supplemented by a complete bibliography of serial extractions so that practitioners may study the steps necessary for successful serial extraction cases. (See *Suggested Readings* at the end of this book.)

The majority of Class III relationships in the primary dentitions are pseudo-Class III and when carefully analyzed they are found to be anterior crossbites. In Chapter 5 the recognition and treatment of anterior cross bites were discussed. Pseudo-Class III occlusal relationships should be followed carefully, since in many cases there is a tendency for the permanent maxillary incisors to erupt lingually and later than the mandibular incisors, and an anterior crossbite in the early mixed dentition may be observed. The anterior crossbites of the mixed dentitions that are pseudo-Class III relationships are readily treated with a microscrew (Fig. 7–1). Inclined planes or acrylic inclined planes cemented on the mandibular incisors are effective in correcting simple anterior crossbites in the mixed dentition.

Occasionally one observes a true Class III relationship, which is usually a familial autosomal dominant characteristic, and which is very difficult to treat. A cephalometric x-ray and a careful family history is always indicated when a true Class III relationship is suspected in the mixed dentition. It is difficult to appraise the severity of the Class III disharmonies in the early mixed dentition. True Class III occlusal disharmonies in the mixed dentition should always be referred to an orthodontist or a practitioner who has had orthodontic training for observation and treatment. In the more severe types of Class III occlusal disharmonies routine orthodontic treatment alone will not suffice. Surgical orthodontics is often the treatment of choice.

Posterior Crossbites

The majority of posterior crossbites of the mixed and permanent dentition are either environmental or functional. They occur as described in the classification of posterior crossbites in the primary dentition (see *Classification* in Chapter 5). They are easily treated with cross-elastics or split plates, or a fixed expansion appliance may be used on both the maxillary and mandibular arches. Occasionally skeletal crossbites are observed in the mixed dentition and are easily distinguished from functional crossbites. In skeletal crossbites, there is involvement of the jaw relationships as well as tooth relationships, whereas in a functional or environmental crossbite, only the tooth relationships are involved.

Premature Loss of Primary Teeth in the Mixed Dentition

It is well known that many occlusal disharmonies result from the premature loss of primary canines and molars. It is interesting to note

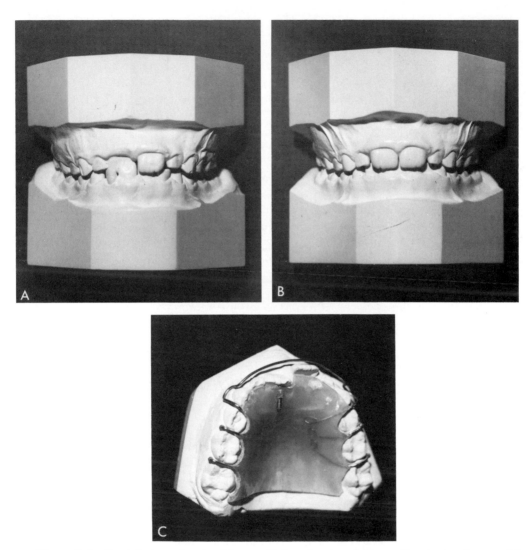

Figure 7–1. Frontal view of casts of 7 year old boy showing right maxillary incisor in cross bite before *(A)* and after *(B)* treatment with a removable appliance and a microscrew. *C*, Removable appliance with ball clasp in place on cast before treatment. Note bite plane lateral to microscrew to open bite and microscrew embedded in removable appliance. (Courtesy of Dr. Leonard J. Carapezza, Wayland, Massachusetts.)

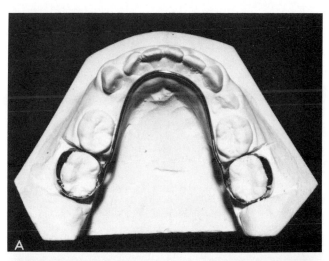

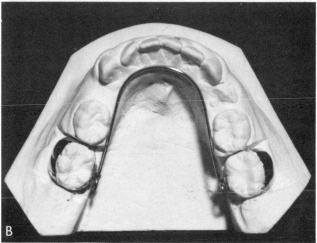

Figure 7–2

A, Fixed soldered passive lingual arch wire (stainless steel, 0.032 or 0.036 in.) for maintaining upright position of first permanent molars and arch space for premolars and canines. Band material (0.005 × 0.180 in.) or preformed molar bands may be used.

B, Removable passive lingual arch wire with loop. This type may be used to maintain space and keep molars in an upright position. The arch wire may be removed and the loop may be activated to move molars distally when additional arch space is necessary. (Courtesy of Rocky Mountain/Orthodontics.)

that when primary maxillary or mandibular incisors are lost early a loss of space rarely occurs. The most important primary teeth for maintaining space for the permanent teeth are the primary canines and first and second primary molars. When primary molars are prematurely lost and the first permanent molar has erupted, a passive lingual arch wire is a simple appliance that will preserve space for the permanent canines and premolars. A passive lingual arch wire may be used on the maxilla and mandible (Fig. 7–2). If the first permanent molar is not fully erupted, care should be taken to adjust the lingual arch wire or remake it as the first permanent molar moves into its full eruptive position (Fig. 7–3). Removable appliances may also be used but they should be used only with a cooperative young patient. Very often primary molars are lost and the children are not seen at regular intervals, and there is a mesial drift of the first permanent molars with loss of space for the premolars. A space regainer may be used to move the first permanent molars distally to their proper position (Figs. 7–4 and 7–5). After the first permanent molar is in its proper position, the space regainer may be fixed and used as a space maintainer.

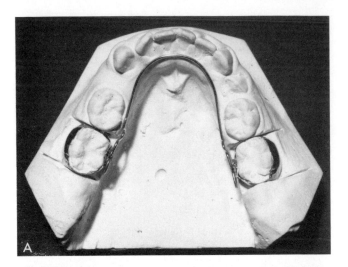

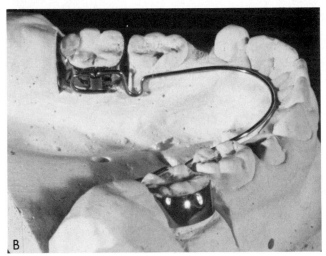

Figure 7–3

A, Removable passive lingual arch wire showing Ellis tube spot-welded to band. Rocky Mountain prefabricated lingual arch is inserted into the Ellis tube.

B, Loop on lingual arch may be activated for expansion, contraction or arch maintenance. (Courtesy of Rocky Mountain/Orthodontics.)

The Denholtz Muscle Anchorage Appliance

The Denholtz appliance is a functional method for muscle development and tooth movement and should be considered a useful auxillary appliance in pediatric dentistry and orthodontic therapy (Figs. 7–6 and 7–7). It has a variety of uses, which may be summarized as follows:

1. The appliance may act as a functional muscle stimulator for hypotonicity of the upper lip and in this way develop a tight lip seal which helps correct mouth breathing. It is useful in open bite cases of environmental origin.

2. In cases of mandibular lip biting the Denholtz lip bumper prevents lip biting by pushing the lower lip out, in this way making it difficult to bite the lower lip.

3. In the primary and mixed dentitions the Denholtz appliance may be used to move the molars distally for satisfactory molar relationships

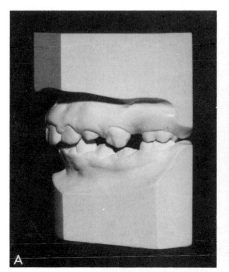
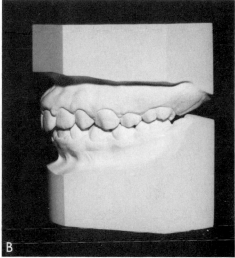

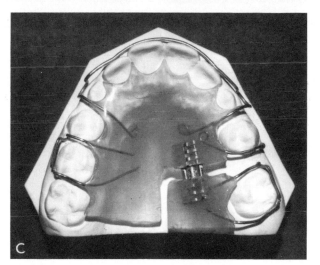

Figure 7–4. Lateral view of casts of 10 year old boy with loss of space for maxillary second premolar before *(A)* and after *(B)* treatment with a double pin expansion screw. *C,* Removable appliance in place on cast. Note labial arch modified Adams clasps and double pin expansion screw. (Courtesy of Dr. Leonard J. Carapezza, Wayland, Massachusetts.)

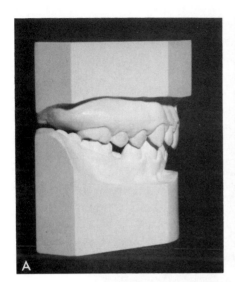
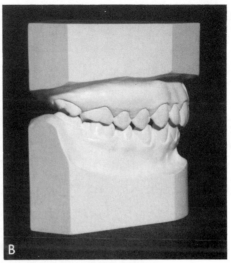
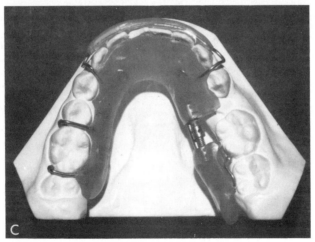

Figure 7–5. Lateral view of casts of an 11 year old with loss of space for mandibular second premolar before *(A)* and after *(B)* treatment with single pin expansion screw. *C,* Removable appliance in place on cast. Note labial arch and ball clasps. (Courtesy of Dr. Leonard J. Carapezza, Wayland, Massachusetts.)

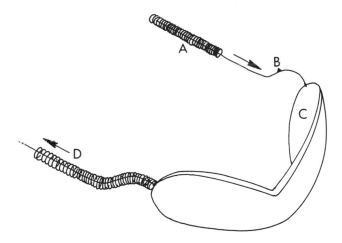

Figure 7–6. Diagrammatic sketch of the basic Denholtz muscle anchorage appliance. Place closed coil *A* over the end section wire until it contacts the screw-on spur *(B)*. Then screw closed coil *A* until it reaches point *C* on the shield portion of the appliance, and open the coil as shown at *D* to activate the appliance. (Courtesy of Rocky Mountain/Orthodontics.)

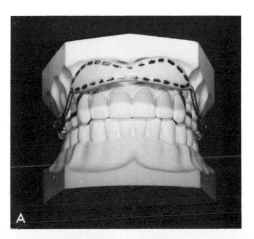

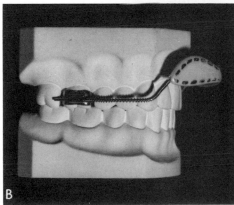

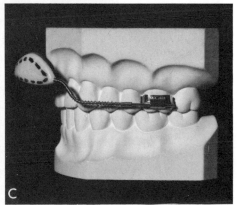

Figure 7–7. Frontal *(A)* and lateral *(B)* views of Denholtz muscle anchorage appliance in place. The dashed lines indicate the final shape of the appliance after it has been rubber-wheeled down to fit high into the mucobuccal fold. (Courtesy of Rocky Mountain/Orthodontics.)

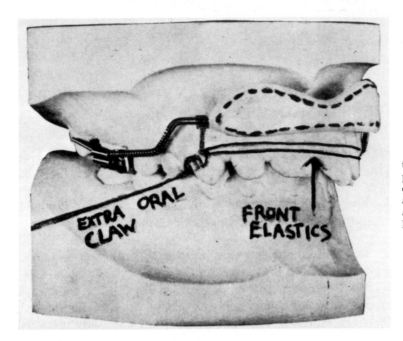

Figure 7–8. Casts showing the Denholtz muscle anchorage appliance in place with an extraoral claw which may be used for elastics across anteriors, cervical traction and Class II elastics. (Courtesy of Rocky Mountain/Orthodontics.)

and is adaptable with extraoral therapy and multibanded techniques (Figs. 7–8 and 7–9).

Prolonged Retention of Primary Teeth

Occlusal disharmonies may be caused by the prolonged retention of primary teeth. When primary teeth are retained beyond their exfoliation time the permanent successors may erupt in malposition, or non-eruption of the succedaneous teeth may occur. In Chapter 5 overretention of primary incisors was discussed. A large number of occlusal disharmonies resulting from prolonged retention of primary teeth can be prevented by systematic roentgenographic examinations and by timely intervention. It is only with the use of roentgenograms that we may determine the extent of resorption of the roots of the primary teeth, atypical resorption and the degree of calcification of the roots of the permanent teeth. Chronological age is of no significance in the diagnosis of prolonged retention, and it should not be used as the criterion for the removal of primary teeth. In some cases of non-eruption due to prolonged retention of primary teeth, calcification of the roots of the permanent teeth may be completed while the overlying primary teeth are still in position. When advanced root calcification occurs in non-erupted permanent teeth, considerable eruption force may be lost so that, following the removal of the overretained primary teeth, the permanent teeth may be retarded in emerging into the oral cavity and space maintenance is often necessary. In some cases eruption may not occur and requires surgical orthodontic intervention.

Removal of overretained primary teeth is an important factor in maintaining occlusal harmony.

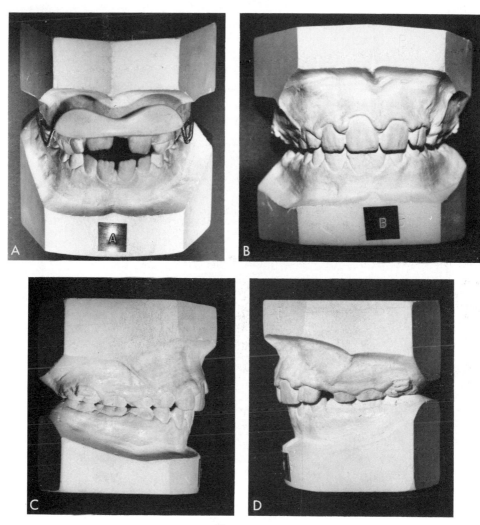

Figure 7–9

A, Frontal view of Denholtz muscle anchorage appliance of patient with mixed dentition and open bite associated with tongue habit, before treatment.

B, Frontal view of same patient 1 year after treatment with muscle anchorage appliance and cervical elastic.

C, D, Lateral views of the same patient. Note double tubes on molar bands. (Courtesy of Rocky Mountain/Orthodontics.)

ORAL HABITS

Epidemiological surveys have shown that approximately 20 per cent of children indulge in oral habits. In the mixed dentition, when such habits persist, there is a severe occlusal disharmony in the anterior part of the mouth. Thumbsucking, tongue thrusting and reverse swallowing habits may accentuate an occlusal disharmony.

If the habit cannot be broken voluntarily, one of the best methods of treatment is either a removable Hawley with a crib (Fig. 7–10) or a fixed appliance with a crib. Children who are tongue thrusters and who have reverse swallowing habits should be referred to a speech therapist. A habit reminder for tongue thrusting and reverse swallowing habits, in conjunction with the sugarless wafer and tongue exercises (see Chapter 5), may reduce the occlusal disharmony in the anterior part of the mouth (Fig. 7–11).

DIASTEMA

A diastema is found in a large majority of children after the permanent central incisors emerge and erupt (Fig. 7–12).

The diastema is temporary, and with the eruption of the permanent lateral incisors into the arch curve, the space between the permanent central incisors usually closes. In some instances one may find a large fibrous frenum with the maxillary permanent incisors in contact and in good alignment. Frena may also be found in association with a diastema.

Occasionally one finds a diastema after the permanent laterals have erupted into the arch curve, in association with a large fibrous frenum. Before surgical removal of the frenum is attempted, roentgenograms of the child should be taken to observe the bone pattern between the central incisors. A true diastema may have a variety of bone patterns which contribute to the space between the permanent central incisors. The parents and siblings of the affected child should be examined, if possible, to observe the occurrence of diastemas in the family. When a diastema occurs as a familial characteristic, it creates a difficult problem in treatment. The central incisors, after they are brought together, very often separate after appliance and retention therapy are completed.

True diastemas should be referred for treatment to an orthodontist or to a practitioner who has had orthodontic training. When a diastema occurs in association with a large fibrous frenum, and the bone pattern between the permanent central incisors appears regular, it may be assumed that the frenum may contribute to the diastema. Before a frenectomy is contemplated, it is essential that the space be closed. Diastema closure may be accomplished with a simple fixed appliance utilizing elastics.

Diastemas may also occur in the mixed dentition in association with hypodontia, supernumerary teeth, mesiodens (Fig. 7–13), peg-shaped laterals and agenesis of the permanent lateral incisors (Fig. 7–14). Habits such as thumbsucking, tongue thrusting, lip biting and lip sucking are capable of producing a diastema between the permanent central incisors.

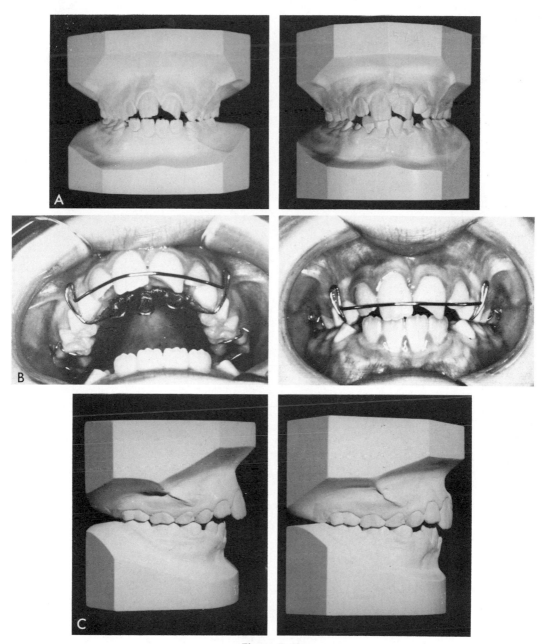

Figure 7-10

A, Anterior view of casts of an 8 year old girl illustrating open bite owing to thumb sucking, before and after wearing removable habit reminder.

B, Habit reminder in place after it was worn diligently for five months.

C, Lateral view of casts before and after wearing habit reminder for five months. Note reduction of open bite.

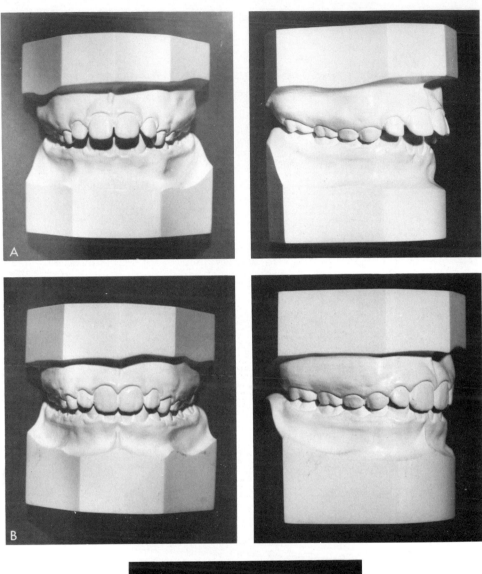

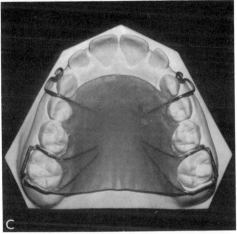

Figure 7–11

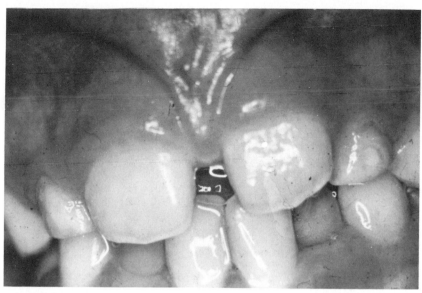

Figure 7–12. Large fibrous frenum between permanent central incisors in a 7 year old child. Note presence of primary laterals.

Postorthodontic relapses of diastemas between the maxillary central incisors create a serious problem and predispose the periodontium to periodontal disease. Numerous treatments have been utilized to hold the central incisors together—for example, the fabrication of interlocking inlays on the mesiolingual aspect of the approximating incisors. These treatments are difficult and at present there is none that will successfully hold the central incisors together.

Recently, Bell (1970) has described a treatment for larger intercisal diastemas in the adult dentition (Fig. 7–15*A*). An osteotomy of the interdental spaces between the apices of the central incisors and the anterior nasal aperture is performed (Fig. 7–15*B*). The dentoalveolar segments are opposed and fixed with wire ligature (Fig. 7–15*C*). The maxillary incisors are banded with an appropriate labial light wire ligation, or a Hawley appliance may be used with wire to approximate the central incisors, (Fig. 7–15*D*). Although this treatment appears successful, long-term observation will determine its permanence (Fig. 7–15*E*). This type of treatment may be considered for the correction of congenital diastemas as well as for relapses of postorthodontic recurrences of diastemas.

Figure 7–11

A, Frontal and lateral views of casts of a 1 year old boy with thumb sucking and tongue thrusting habits, before treatment with an elastic hook retainer and acrylic tongue guard.

B, Frontal and lateral views of casts after patient had worn appliance for 10 months.

C, Removable appliance on cast. Note tongue-guard hooks for elastics to retract anterior teeth. Modified Adams clasps.

(Courtesy of Dr. Leonard J. Carapezza, Wayland, Massachusetts.)

See illustration on opposite page.

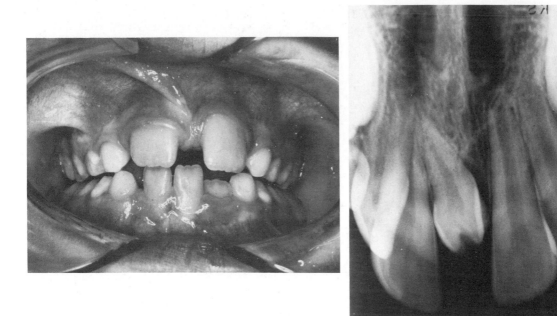

Figure 7–13. Diastemas in an 8 year old girl resulting from a mesiodens.

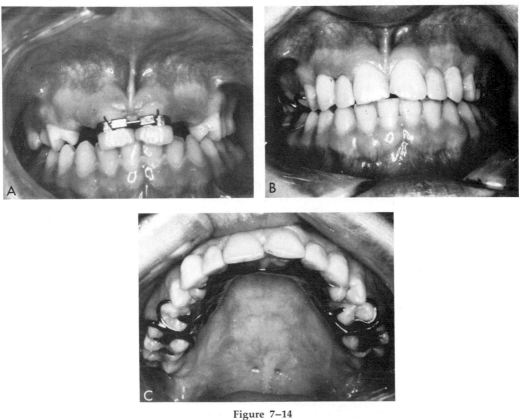

Figure 7–14

A, A diastema closure utilizing Johnson orthodontic bands with flat wire in brackets and caps on brackets. Patient had a large diastma owing to absence of permanent laterals and canines.

B, Frontal view of stainless steel partial denture in position after central incisors were moved into their proper position in the arch.

C, Palatal view of partial denture in place.

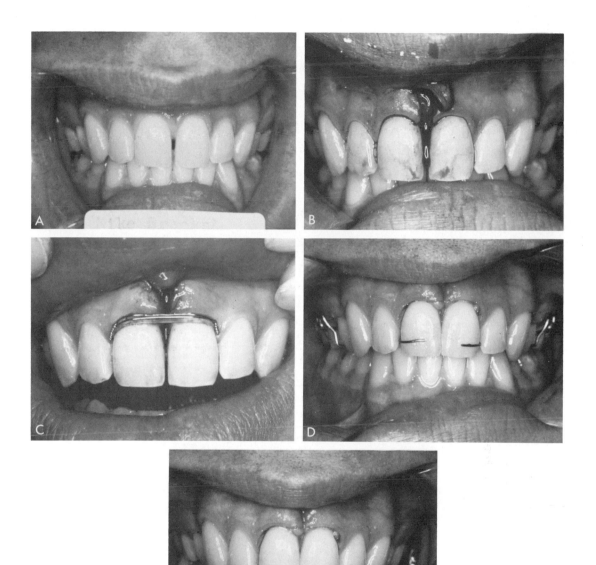

Figure 7–15

A, Frontal view of diastema in a 22 year old male before osteotomy.

B, Frontal view after osteotomy.

C, Dentoalveolar segment opposed and fixed with wire ligatures.

D, Hawley appliance with light wire on distal of centrals to approximate central incisors.

E, Frontal view of mouth a month after osteotomy.

ECTOPIC ERUPTION

Ectopic eruptions of the first permanent molars may occur either in the maxillary or in the mandibular arch (Fig. 7–16 *A, B*). Other permanent teeth may erupt ectopically (Fig. 7–16*C*), but the first permanent molars are the teeth most frequently affected. Such eruptions may be unilateral or bilateral, and the most frequent site is in the maxillary arch. They may be observed as early as ages 3 to 3½ years. If the child is seen early, and the first permanent molar has not drifted too far mesially, a No. 23 gauge brass ligature wire is threaded between the maxillary first permanent molar and the second primary molar, and the ends are twisted with pliers. The wedging of the brass wire will move the first molar distally, relieve the impaction and allow for the emergence and eruption of the maxillary second premolar. If the child is seen when the first permanent molar has emerged and erupted, and has partially blocked out the second premolar, headgear may be used to move the molar or molars distally. After the molars are brought into their proper position, a lingual arch wire is placed to maintain arch length.

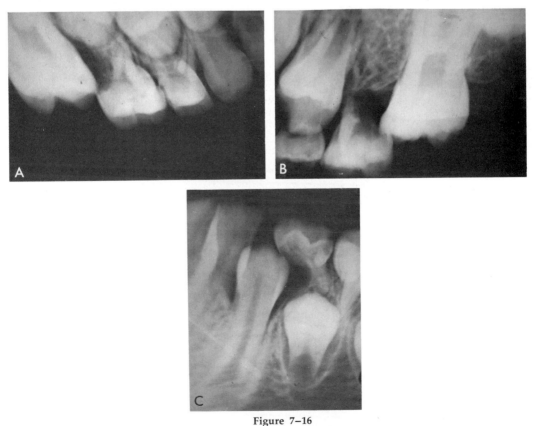

Figure 7–16

A, B, Ectopic eruption of maxillary first permanent molars.
C, Ectopic eruption of mandibular canine.
(Courtesy of Dr. Joseph Keller, New York, N.Y.)

ANKYLOSIS

In the mixed dentition, when the ankylosed teeth are 2 mm. or more below the occlusal plane of the adjacent teeth, extractions are indicated. Allowing these teeth to remain will cause mesial and distal drifting of the adjacent teeth and displacement of the unerupted permanent tooth follicles (Fig. 7–17).

The longer an ankylosed tooth remains in the mouth, the more difficult it is to extract it because of absence of the periodontal ligament and subsequent firm attachment to the alveolar bone. After the teeth are removed, either fixed or removable appliances may be employed to maintain the space.

AGENESIS

It has been shown that in the congenital absence of third molars, there is a size reduction of the remaining teeth. From various epidemiological reports the permanent teeth most frequently missing, other than the third molar, are the maxillary lateral incisors and the mandibular second premolars. In a study of agenesis in the permanent dentition, Baum and Cohen (1971a, b, c; 1973) have shown that when permanent laterals or premolars are missing there is an even greater size reduction of the remaining teeth (Fig. 7–18). In children who have permanent lateral incisors and second premolars missing, the teeth are smaller than those found in the general population, and there is a high incidence of Class II occlusal disharmonies. When maxillary permanent lateral incisors are absent bilaterally, there is usually a diastema between the maxillary central incisors. The diastema may be treated with flat wire and brackets, and latex elastics may be used to bring the central incisors together (Fig. 7–14).

After the central incisors are in contact, a removable appliance may be made to replace the missing lateral incisors. Fixed prosthesis should be delayed until the child is at least 18 years or older. Occasionally, if the two central incisors are large, they may be brought together with a small diastema between them and the canines may be moved into the arch curve so that there is a small diastema between the mesial surface of the canine and the distal surface of the central incisor (Fig. 7–19). When the patient is 16 years or older, the canines may be ground on their incisal edges to improve esthetic appearance.

In multiple agenesis, simple fixed appliances are used to bring permanent central incisors together, and removable appliances are used for esthetic improvement. In many cases of agenesis the primary teeth are without permanent successors. It is wise to extract the primary teeth and in their place fabricate a temporary acrylic partial denture which will serve the child functionally and esthetically until he or she is older, and then a permanent prosthesis may be fabricated.

In the treatment of agenesis of permanent teeth, treatment is always a compromise, since in most instances the teeth are smaller and there is a high incidence of Class II occlusal disharmony. Children with agenesis are very conscious of their condition, and if the practitioner can construct a

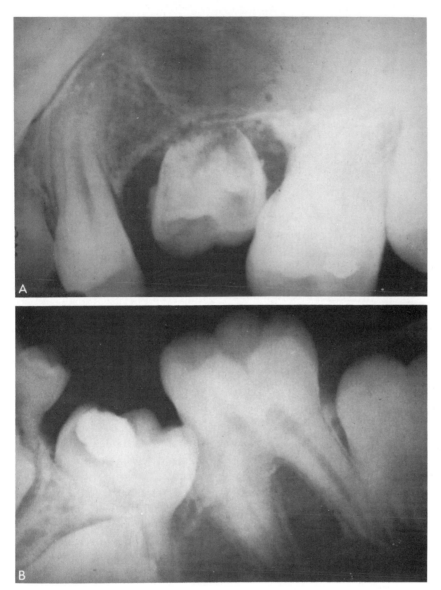

Figure 7–17

A, Ankylosed maxillary second primary molar with absence of second premolar. Ankylosed mandibular second primary molar.

B, Note mesial drift of first permanent molar.

(Courtesy of Dr. Joseph Keller, New York, N.Y.)

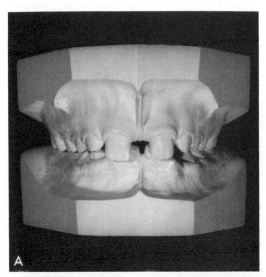

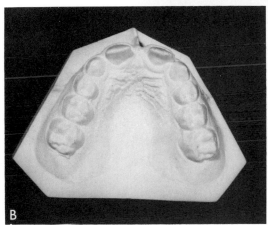

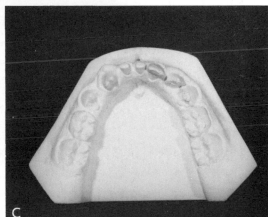

Figure 7–18

  A, Multiple agenesis in mixed dentition of 9 year old girl. Note small teeth and closed bite and tendency for a Class II occlusal relationship.

  B,C, Occlusal views.

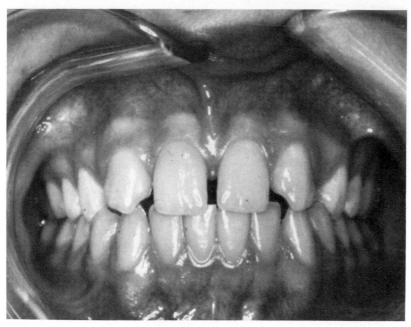

Figure 7–19. Sixteen year old girl with congenital absence of maxillary laterals. Central incisors approximated with a removable appliance and canines guided into arch with a Hawley removable appliance.

prosthesis that is pleasing, harmonious and well functional with the remaining teeth, the child will accept this gratefully, and it will have a profound effect on his general well-being (Fig. 7–20).

TREATMENT FOR MANDIBULAR INCISOR CROWDING

Recent studies by Peck and Peck have shown that satisfactory, well aligned mandibular incisors are reduced in size mesiodistally and are increased in size faciolingually. From these observations irregularities involving the mesiodistal and faciolingual dimensions of the mandibular incisors contribute to crowding in the mandibular incisor region. Peck and Peck have proposed an index which incorporates both the mesiodistal and faciolingual diameters of the mandibular incisors, as follows:

$$\text{Index} = \frac{\text{Mesiodistal (MD) crown diameter in mm.}}{\text{Faciolingual (FL) crown diameter in mm.}} \times 100$$

This index is referred to as the *MD/FL index* and is a numerical expression of crown shape of the mandibular incisors as viewed incisally.

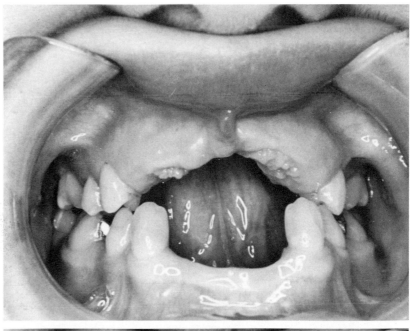

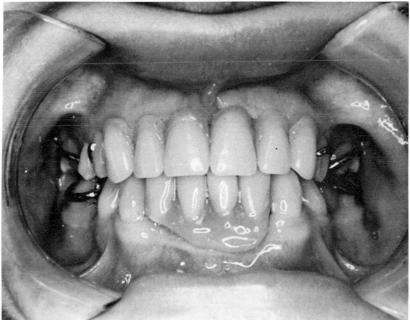

Figure 7–20. Fourteen year old girl with multiple permanent tooth agenesis and deformity of the maxilla before prostheses were inserted. Maxillary and mandibular prostheses in place.

The Clinical Application

The observed relationship between mandibular incisor shape and the presence and absence of mandibular incisor crowding has significant clinical relevance. The MD/FL index as previously described and utilized is a numerical expression of crown shape. As such, it provides an effective clinical method for diagnosing tooth shape deviations which influence and contribute to mandibular incisor crowding.

Clinical Principles

In order to recognize tooth shape deviations, a knowledge of optimum tooth shape is necessary. For the mandibular incisors, the lower the MD/FL index, the more favorable the tooth shape relative to good alignment. Our studies have shown that well aligned mandibular central incisors have an MD/FL index of 88.4 ±

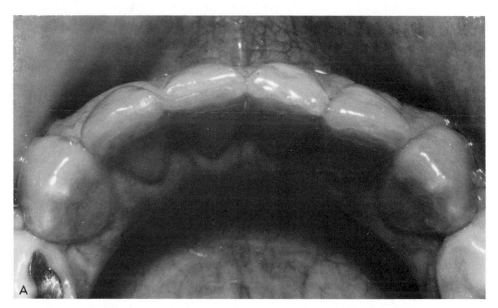

Tooth	MD	FL	MD/FL Index	MD/FL Index Standards
2⌐	5.3	6.4	83	90 – 95
1⌐	5.2	5.8	90	88 – 92
⌐1	5.2	5.7	91	88 – 92
⌐2	5.5	6.3	87	90 – 95

Figure 7–21

A, Photographs of the mandibular incisors of an orthodontically untreated individual. Well aligned mandibular incisors that are well within the MD/FL (mesiodistal/faciolingual) index standards.

4.3, while well-aligned mandibular lateral incisors have an index of 90.4 ± 4.8 (Fig. 7–21*A*).

From these data we have adapted the clinical standards which we use in determining whether a lower incisor is favorably or unfavorably shaped relative to good alignment. The following ranges are employed as *clinical guidelines for the maximum limit of desirable MD/FL index values for the lower incisors:*

Mandibular central incisor	88–92
Mandibular lateral incisor	90–95

The lower limit of each range represents approximately the mean value of the MD/FL index of well-aligned teeth. The upper limit of each range is derived from the lower limit plus one standard deviation.

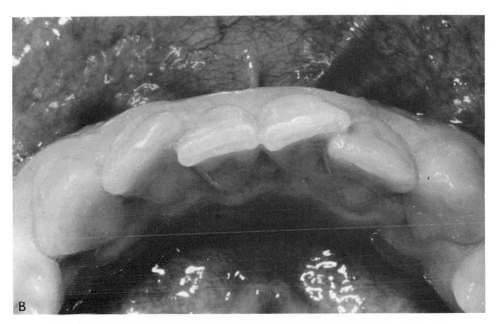

Tooth	MD	FL	MD/FL Index	MD/FL Index Standards
2⌐	5.8	5.9	98	90 – 95
1⌐	5.4	5.3	101	88 – 92
⌐1	5.2	5.4	96	88 – 92
⌐2	6.3	5.6	111	90 – 95

Figure 7–21 *Continued.* *B,* Patient with mandibular incisor crowding, showing a higher MD/FL index than desirable MD/FL index standards.

(From Peck, S., and Peck, H.: Orthodontic Aspects of Dental Anthropology. Angle Ort. ed., 45:95–102, 1975.)

Lower incisors within or below these ranges are considered favorably shaped. Any lower incisor with an MD/FL index above these ranges however, is considered to have a crown shape deviation which may influence or contribute to the crowding phenomenon (Fig. 7–21*B*).

Of course, this is not always the case. Since we are dealing with four teeth when we speak of mandibular incisor crowding, good alignment is often present with various combinations of favorably and unfavorably shaped teeth. For instance, lateral incisors with an index of 97 may be well aligned in a mandibular arch with central incisors that have an index of 86.

However, an MD/FL index in excess of 100 for any of the lower incisors represents a severe shape deviation, characteristic of existing or potential tooth irregularity (Fig. 7–21*B*). From a previously described control population sample, we have estimated that approximately 15 per cent of the population have an MD/FL index greater than 100 for one or both mandibular central incisors. Similarly, about 25 per cent of the population have mandibular lateral incisors with an MD/FL index in excess of 100. The average orthodontic practice contains a high concentration of these persons. They usually are the patients exhibiting bimaxillary crowding.

Patients whose mandibular incisors have MD/FL indices above the desired range may well be candidates for the removal of some mesial and/or distal tooth substance in conjunction with orthodontic therapy. This procedure is commonly called "stripping." Although part of the orthodontic vernacular, "stripping" is a somewhat distasteful term. Articles and texts frequently resort to euphemisms, such as "proximal reduction." We are convinced that purposeful tooth size alteration will have an increasingly significant place in the orthodontist's therapeutic armamentarium. It is therefore deserving of a more exacting, more appropriate name. In place of "stripping" we propose "reproximation" a word whose derivation implies "the act of 'redoing' the approximal surfaces." . . . By definition, *tooth reproximation is a clinical procedure involving the reduction, anatomic recontouring, and protection of the mesial and/or distal enamel surfaces of a permanent tooth.* Protection in this instance refers to the topical application of cariostatic agents, such as acidulated phosphate-fluoride.

Clinical Methods

The mesiodistal (MD) and faciolingual (FL) crown diameters of the mandibular incisor teeth are measured directly in the mouth, not on plaster casts. The maximum MD diameter is usually located at or near the incisal edge (Fig. 7–22*A*), while the maximum FL diameter is found almost always beneath the gingival margin, thus precluding the use of plaster casts (Fig. 7–22*B*).

Measurements are taken with a millimeter caliper calibrated at least to tenths of a millimeter. Some calipers have a vernier scale (the Boley gauge, for example) for reading out the measurements, while others have a dial scale. For tooth measurements, where tenths of a millimeter are important, we prefer a dial caliper because of its superior readability and precision. The caliper tips must be specially sharpened to a knife-edged point to make accurate measuring possible.

We take the lower incisor measurements in a sequence, beginning with the four MD measurements, right lateral incisor to left lateral incisor, followed by the four FL measurements, right lateral incisor to left lateral incisor. The accuracy of each measurement is quickly checked by comparing the values recorded for the right lateral incisor with those of the left lateral incisor and making the same comparisons for the central incisors. Any gross discrepancy observed between right and left measurements often is a sign that a measurement error was made, since right and left tooth dimensions usually correspond closely. In these cases the measurements in question are routinely repeated, even though gross asymmetries in crown dimension are not uncommon.

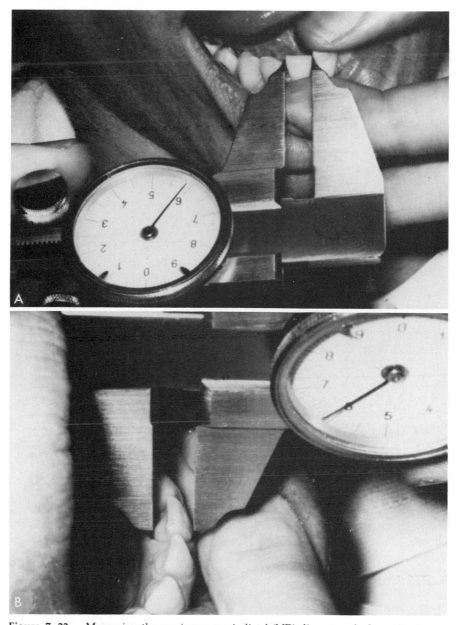

Figure 7–22. Measuring the maximum mesiodistal (MD) diameter of a lower incisor.

A, A dial caliper is employed. The caliper beaks are positioned near the incisal edge and are held perpendicular to the long axis of the tooth.

B, Measuring the maximum faciolingual (FL) diameter of a lower incisor. The dial caliper beaks are slipped slightly beneath the gingival margin and are held parallel to the long axis of the tooth.

(From Peck, H., and Peck, S.: An index for assessing tooth shape deviations as applied to the mandibular incisors. Am. J. Orthod., *61*:384–401, 1972.)

The MD and FL crown measurements are recorded in an approximate table or grid. The next step is to compute the MD/FL indices of the four teeth measured.

This procedure is simplified with the use of a mathematical reference table developed for this purpose (Table 7–1). The reference table provides the computed value of the MD/FL index values from 86 to 119. All values below 86 are exceedingly favorable and therefore require no further clinical consideration. Values above 119 are exceedingly unfavorable but occur very rarely. (From Peck and Peck, 1972.)

When reproxima ion is indicated, abrasive steel strips are used to reduce the interproximal enamel (Fig. 7–23A) and provide access for an abrasive steel disc used in conjunction with a disc-guard (Fig. 7–23B). Anatomical recontouring of the tooth is then completed with green stones and polishing strips (Fig. 7–23C). Acidulated phosphate-fluoride is then applied to the recontoured teeth for protection of the enamel (Fig. 7–23D).

MESIODISTAL (MD) CROWN DIMENSION — rows: FACIOLINGUAL (FL) CROWN DIMENSION

FL \ MD	4.2	4.3	4.4	4.5	4.6	4.7	4.8	4.9	5.0	5.1	5.2	5.3	5.4	5.5	5.6	5.7	5.8	5.9	6.0	6.1	6.2	6.3	6.4	6.5	6.6	6.7	6.8	6.9	7.0	7.1	7.2	7.3	7.4
4.7	89	91	94	96	98	100	102	104	106	109	111	113	115	117	119																		
4.8	88	90	92	94	96	98	100	102	104	106	108	110	112	115	117	119																	
4.9	86	88	90	92	94	96	98	100	102	104	106	108	110	112	114	116	118																
5.0		86	88	90	92	94	96	98	100	102	104	106	108	110	112	114	116	118															
5.1			86	88	90	92	94	96	98	100	102	104	106	108	110	112	114	116	118														
5.2				87	88	90	92	94	96	98	100	102	104	106	108	110	112	113	115	117	119												
5.3					87	89	91	92	94	96	98	100	102	104	106	108	109	111	113	115	117	119											
5.4						87	89	91	93	94	96	98	100	102	104	106	107	109	111	113	115	117	119										
5.5							87	89	91	93	95	96	98	100	102	104	105	107	109	111	113	115	116	118									
5.6							86	88	89	91	93	95	96	98	100	102	104	105	107	109	111	112	114	116	118								
5.7								86	88	89	91	93	95	96	98	100	102	104	105	107	109	111	112	114	116	118	119						
5.8									86	88	90	91	93	95	97	98	100	102	103	105	107	109	110	112	114	116	117	119					
5.9										86	88	90	92	93	95	97	98	100	102	103	105	107	108	110	112	114	115	117	119				
6.0											87	88	90	92	93	95	97	98	100	102	103	105	107	108	110	112	113	115	117	118			
6.1												87	89	90	92	93	95	97	98	100	102	103	105	107	108	110	111	113	115	116	118		
6.2													87	89	90	92	94	95	97	98	100	102	103	105	106	108	110	111	113	115	116	118	119
6.3													86	87	89	90	92	94	95	97	98	100	102	103	105	106	108	110	111	113	114	116	117
6.4														86	88	89	91	92	94	95	97	98	100	102	103	105	106	108	109	111	112	114	116
6.5															86	88	89	91	92	94	95	97	98	100	102	103	105	106	108	109	111	112	114
6.6																86	88	89	91	92	94	95	97	98	100	102	103	105	106	108	109	111	112
6.7																	87	88	90	91	93	94	96	97	99	100	101	103	104	106	107	109	110
6.8																		87	88	90	91	93	94	96	97	99	100	101	103	104	106	107	109
6.9																			87	88	90	91	93	94	96	97	99	100	101	103	104	106	107
7.0																				87	89	90	91	93	94	96	97	99	100	101	103	104	106
7.1																					87	89	90	92	93	94	96	97	99	100	101	103	104
7.2																					86	88	89	90	92	93	94	96	97	99	100	101	103
7.3																						86	88	89	90	92	93	95	96	97	99	100	101
7.4																							86	88	89	91	92	93	95	96	97	99	100
7.5																								87	88	89	91	92	93	95	96	97	99

(From Peck, H., and Peck, S.: An index for assessing tooth shape deviations as applied to the mandibular incisors. Am. J. Orthod., *61*:384–401, 1972.)

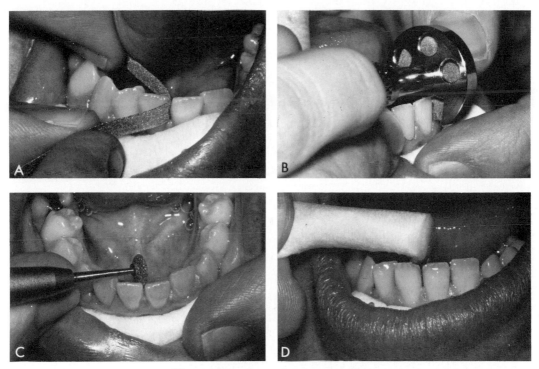

Figure 7–23. Reproximation methods.

A, Enamel reduction with abrasive steel strips.

B, Enamel reduction using safe-sided abrasive steel discs with special disc guard.

C, Anatomical recontouring with fine white or green stone.

D, Application of acidulated phosphate-fluoride to ground enamel surfaces.

(From Peck, H., and Peck, S.: Reproximation (enamel stripping) as an essential orthodontic treatment ingredient. Transactions of the Third International Orthodontic Congress, London, pp. 513–523, 1975.)

The MD/FL Index in Clinical Diagnosis

To illustrate the clinical application of the MD/FL index as a means of detecting and evaluating tooth shape deviations of the mandibular incisors, two diagnostic cases will be presented.

DIAGNOSTIC CASE 1.   All four lower incisors of this patient show extreme tooth shape deviations (Fig. 7–24). The right and left lateral incisors have MD/FL indices of 119 and 112, respectively. The right and left central incisors have MD/FL indices of 102 and 103, respectively. There is marked crowding, for which the untoward shape and size of the lower incisors are at least partly responsible. As part of this patient's orthodontic treatment (which in this case calls for premolar extractions), reproximation of the four mandibular incisors is mandatory. Otherwise, recrowding of the lower anterior teeth will surely follow retention.

The lateral incisors are so severely deviated that reproximation, limited by the thickness of the mesial and distal enamel, can only lessen the deviations rather than eliminate them completely. For the central incisors, however, we may expect that reproximation will yield favorable MD/FL indices.

With tooth shape deviations of the intensity observed in these incisors, we would expect a total of 2 to 3 mm. of mesiodistal enamel to be removed by reproximation. A loss of tooth substance of this magnitude may upset the maxillary to mandibular anterior tooth size ratio. Therefore, selective reproximation of the mandibular incisors may also be indicated to maintain a harmonious anterior intermaxillary relationship. This case represents extreme tooth shape deviations, requiring reproximation of the lower incisors as an integral part of orthodontic therapy. (From Peck and Peck, 1972.)

DIAGNOSTIC CASE 2. The second patient had crowding of mandibular incisors with high MD/FL index values before reproximation (Fig. 7–25*A*). Figure 7–25*B*, shows the same patient after reproximation. Alignment of mandibular incisors was carried out with a removable Hawley labial arch appliance (Fig. 7–25*C*).

Clinical procedures for tooth size analysis of the mandibular incisors have been introduced by Peck and Peck based upon the MD/FL index. In postorthodontic cases when there is crowding of the mandibular incisors, this method is useful. It also may be used in the permanent dentition when there is a satisfactory occlusal relationship with moderate to severe crowding of the mandibular incisors.

This diagnostic analysis and the reproximation procedure are valuable as part of comprehensive orthodontic therapy and when mandibular incisor crowding is observed in patients who have a satisfactory posterior occlusal relationship.

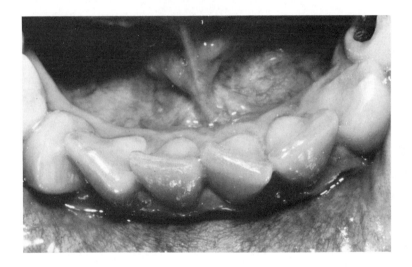

Tooth	MD	FL	MD/FL Index	MD/FL Index Standards
2⌐	7.0	5.9	119	90 – 95
1⌐	5.8	5.7	102	88 – 92
⌐1	6.0	5.8	103	88 – 92
⌐2	6.7	6.0	112	90 – 95

Figure 7–24. Patient with marked mandibular incisor crowding and associated severe irregularity of tooth morphology. (From Peck, H., and Peck, S.: An index for assessing tooth shape deviations as applied to the mandibular incisors. Am. J. Orthod., *61*:384–401, 1972.)

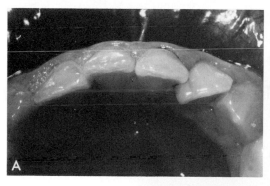

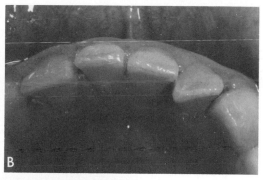

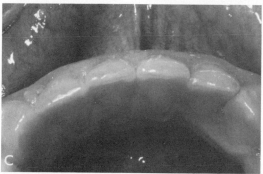

TOOTH	MD	FL	50% ENAMEL Thickness	ORIG MD/FL	DESIRED			ACHIEVED		
					MD/FL	MD	REPROX	MD/FL	MD	REPROX
2⌐	6.8	5.8	1.0	117	100	5.8	1.0	100	5.8	1.0
1⌐	6.0	6.0	.8	100	88	5.3	.7	90	5.4	.6
⌐1	5.9	5.9	.7	100	88	5.2	.7	92	5.4	.5
⌐2	6.8	6.1	1.0	111	95	5.8	1.0	95	5.8	1.0
D							3.4			3.1

Figure 7–25

A, Patient with high MD/FL index values before reproximation.
B, After reproximation.
C, Alignment of mandibular incisors employing a removable Hawley labial arch appliance.
D, Peck and Peck analysis forms with recorded MD/FL index before and after reproximation.
(Courtesy of Drs. Sheldon and Harvey Peck, Boston, Massachusetts.)

REFERENCES

Space Maintainance

Barber, T. K.: The concept of preventive orthodontics. J. Dent. Child., *33*:75–86, 1966.
Bunch, W. B.: Space maintenance using the lingual arch. Dent. Clin. N. Am., pp. 489–498, July, 1966.
Cohen, M. M.: Prophylactic orthodontics and tooth guidance. III. Dent. J., *26*:707–716, 815–820, 1957.
Daugherty, C. W.: Mixed dentition guidance. S. Carolina Dent. J., *28*:4–13, 1970.
Easlick, K. A.: Management of spaces during the period of the primary and mixed dentitions. An introduction to the problems. J. N.J. State Dent. Soc., *31*:9–10, 1960.

Fanning, E. A.: Effect of extraction of deciduous molars on the formation and eruption of their successors. Angle Orthod., *32*:44–53, 1962.

Fogels, H. R., and Shiere, F. R.: A functional space maintainer and guide for the unerupted first permanent molar. J. Dent. Child., *22*:44–47, 1955.

Harris, J.: Restoring mandibular arch length in the mixed and early permanent dentition. Am. J. Orthod., *62*:606–622, 1972.

Kohn, S. I.: Space maintenance. Dent. Clin. N. Am., pp. 703–721, November, 1961.

Kronfeld, S. M., and Addelston, H. K.: Cast space maintainers. J. N.J. State Dent. Soc., *25*:16–21, 1954.

MacLaughlin, J. A., Fogels, H. R., and Shiere, F. R.: The influence of premature primary molar extraction on bicuspid eruption. J. Dent. Child., *34*:399–405, 1967.

Mershon, J. V.: The removable lingual arch appliance. Int. J. Orthod., *12*:1002, 1926.

Ryan, K. J.: Understanding and use of space maintenance procedures. J. Dent. Child., *31*:22–25, 1964.

Schacter, J. J.: Adjustable space maintainer for the general practitioner. J.A.D.A., *66*:817–820, 1963.

Crossbite

Adamson, K. T.: The problem of impacted teeth in orthodontics. Aust. Dent. J., *56*:74–84, 1952.

Cheney, E.: The influence of dentofacial asymmetrics upon treatment procedures. Am. J. Orthod., *38*:934–945, 1952.

Cheney, E.: Indications and methods for the interception of functional crossbites and interlocking. Dent. Clin. N. Am., pp. 385–401, July, 1959.

Clifford, F. O.: Crossbite correction in the deciduous dentition: Principles and procedures. Am. J. Orthod., *59*:343–349, 1971.

Hackel, J. L.: Spontaneous correction of primary anterior tooth in crossbite. J. Dent. Child., *34*:128–129, 1967.

Higley, L. B.: Crossbite—mandibular malposition. J. Dent. Child., *35*:221–223, 1968.

Kutin, G., and Hawes, R. S.: Posterior crossbite in deciduous and mixed dentitions. Am. J. Orthod., *56*:491–504, 1969.

Leighton, B. C.: The early development of crossbites. Dent. Pract., *17*:145–152, 1966.

Moore, J. R., and Hughes, B. O.: Familial factors in diagnosis, treatment and prognosis of dentofacial disturbances. Am. J. Orthod. Oral Surg., *28*:603–639, 1942.

Stoneking, J. L., Barber, T. K., and Lauterstein, A.: Cephalometric analysis of incisor crossbite correction. J. Dent. Child., *32*:3–11, 1965.

Suematsu, H.: Orofiles of patients with anterior crossbite and the changes following orthodontic treatment—roentgenocephalometric study. J. Jap. Orthod. Soc., *27*:248–267, 1968.

Valentine, F., and Howitt, J. W.: Multiplication of early anterior crossbite correction. J. Dent. Child., *37*:76–83, 1970.

Webber, D. L.: The general practitioner's role in the treatment of anterior crossbite. J. Dent. Child., *33*:324–330, 1966.

Wright, C.: Crossbites and their management. Angle Orthod., *23*:35–45, 1953.

Oral Habits

Ayers, W. A., and Gale, E. N.: Psychology and thumbsucking. J.A.D.A., *80*:1335–1337, 1970.

Bakwin, H.: Thumb and finger sucking in children. J. Pediat., *32*:99–101, 1948.

Bakwin, H.: Child behavior and the dentist. J. New Jersey State Dent. Soc., *32*:13–23, 1961.

Barrett, R. H.: One approach to deviate swallowing. Am. J. Orthod., *47*:726, 1961.

Benjamin, L. S.: The beginning of thumbsucking. Child Develop., *30*:1965, 1967.

Bowdon, B. A.: A longitudinal study of the effects of digit and dummy sucking. Am. J. Orthod., *52*:887–901, 1966.

Calisti, L. J. P., Cohen, M. M., and Fales, M. H.: Correlation between malocclusion, oral habits and socio-economic level of pre-school children. J. Dent. Res., *39*:450–454, 1960.

Davidson, P. O., Haryett, R. D., Sandilands, M., and Hansen, F. C.: Thumbsucking: Habit or Symptom? J. Dent. Child., *34*:252–259, 1967.

Fastlight, S.: Dental malocclusion caused by pressure of the tongue and open bite. G.A.C. Med. Mex., *99*:26–33, 1969.

Gale, E. N., and Ayer, A.: Thumbsucking revisited. Am. J. Orthod., *55*:165–170, 1969.

Hansen, M. L., Barnard, L. W., and Case, J. L.: Tongue thrust in pre-school children. Am. J. Orthod., *56*:60–69, 1969.

Hansen, M. L., Hilton, L. M., Barnard, L. W., and Case, J. L.: Tongue thrust in pre-school children. III. Cinefluorographic analysis. Am. J. Orthod., *58*:268–275, 1970.

Hansen, M. L., Barnard, L. W., and Case, J. L.: Tongue thrust in pre-school children. II. Dental occlusal patterns. Am. J. Orthod., *57*:15–22, 1970.

Hansen, L. H., and Cohen, M. S.: Effects of form and function on swallowing and the developing dentition. Am. J. Orthod., *64*:63–82, 1973.

Haryett, R. D., Hansen, F. C., Davidson, P. O., and Sandilands, M. L.: Chronic thumbsucking: the psychological effects and the relative effectiveness of various methods of treatment. Am. J. Orthod., *53*:569–595, 1967.

Haryett, R. D., Hansen, F. C., and Davidson, P. O.: Chronic thumbsucking—a second report on treatment and its psychological effects. Am. J. Orthod., *57*:165–167, 1970.

Hemley, S., and Kronfeld, S. M.: Habits. Dent. Clin. N. Am., pp. 687–701, November, 1961.

Kaplan, M.: A note on the psychological implications of thumbsucking. J. Pediat., *37*:555–560, 1950.

Klein, E. T.: The thumbsucking habit: meaningful or empty? Am. J. Orthod., *59*:283–289, 1971.

Massler, M., and Malone, A. J.: Nail-biting. A review. J. Orthod., *36*:351–367, 1950.

Miller, H.: A treatment procedure for early occlusal disharmonies caused by noxious habits. J.A.D.A., *79*:361–367, 1969.

Nadda, R. S., Khan, I., and Anand, R.: Effect of oral habits on the occlusion in pre-school children. J. Dent. Child., *39*:449–452, 1972.

Norton, L. A., and Gellin, N. E.: Management of digital sucking and tongue thrusting in children. Dent. Clin. N. Am., pp. 363–382, July, 1968.

Porter, D. R.: Implications and interrelations of oral habits. J. Dent. Child., *31*:165–170, 1964.

Rasmus, R. L., and Jacobs, R. M.: Mouth breathing and malocclusion: Quantitative technic for measurement of oral and nasal air-flow velocities. Angle Orthod., *39*:296–299, 1969.

Stansell, B. J.: Effects of deglutition and speech training on dental overjet. J. S. Calif. Dent. Ass., *36*:423–437, 1970.

Straub, W.: Malfunctions of the tongue. I. Am. J. Orthod., *46*:404, 1960.

Tewari, A.: Abnormal oral habits relationship with malocclusion and influence on anterior teeth. J. Indian Dent. Ass., *42*:81–84, 1970.

Tsaltas, G.: Etiology, prognosis and treatment planning of anterior open bites. Acta Stomat. Hellen., *13*:94–101, 1969.

Vasilev, P.: A case of open occlusion due to parafunction of the tongue. Stomatologia, *50*:141–144, 1966.

Whitman, C. L.: Habits can mean trouble. Am. J. Orthod., *37*:647–661, 1951.

Whitman, C. L.: Correction of oral habits. Dent. Clin. N. Am., pp. 541–547, July, 1964.

Diastema—Frenum

Bell, W. H.: Surgical orthodontic treatment of interincisal diastemas. Am. J. Orthod., *57*:158–163, 1970.

Bishara, S. E.: Management of diastemas in orthodontics. Am. J. Orthod., *61*:55–63, 1972.

Ceremello, P. J.: The superior labial frenum and the midline diastema and their relationship to growth and development of the oral structures. Am. J. Orthod., *39*:120–139, 1953.

Dewel, B. F.: Contraindications for surgical resection of the maxillary labial frenum. Dent. Dig., *50*:254–256; 306–311, 1944.

Dewel, B. F.: The normal and abnormal labial frenum. Clinical differentiation. J.A.D.A., *33*:318–329, 1946.

Highley, L. B.: Maxillary labial frenum and midline diastema. J. Dent. Child., *36*:413–414, 1969.

Sanin, C., Seckiguchi, T., and Savara, B. S.: A clinical method for the prediction of closure of the central diastema. J. Dent. Child., *36*:415–418, 1969.

Taylor, J. E.: Clinical observations relating to the normal and abnormal frenum labii superioris. Am. J. Orthod., *25*:646–650, 1939.

West, E. E.: Diastema—a cause for concern. Dent. Clin. N. Am., pp. 425–434, July, 1968.

Ectopic Eruption

Byrd, W. M.: Prevalence of ectopic eruption of the permanent teeth in children between five and ten years of age. Am. J. Orthod., *42*:153, 1956.

Dixon, D. A.: Impactions of first permanent molars. Brit. Dent. J., *106*:281–283, 1959.

Herman, E.: The malposed first permanent molar. New York Dent. J., *35*:343–350, 1969.

Lewis, S. J.: Ectopic eruption of permanent teeth as a factor in premature loss of deciduous teeth. J.A.D.A., *23*:1019–1027, 1936.

Nikiforuk, G.: Ectopic eruption: discussion and clinical report. J. Ontario Dent. A., *25*:241–246, 1948.

O'Meara, W. F.: Ectopic eruption pattern in selected permanent teeth. J. Dent. Res., *41*:607–616, 1962.

Pulver, F.: Etiology and prevalence of ectopic eruption of maxillary first permanent molar. J. Dent. Child., *35*:138–146, 1968.

Ankylosis

Biederman, W.: Ankylosis. Ann. Dent., *12*:1–15, 1953.

Biederman, W.: The problems of the ankylosed tooth. Dent. Clin. N. Am., pp. 409–424, July, 1968.

Breadley, L. J., and McKibben, D. H.: Ankylosis of primary molar teeth. I. Prevalence and characteristics. II. A longitudinal study. J. Dent. Child., *40*:54–63, 1973.

Darling, A. I., and Levers, B. G.: Submerged human deciduous molars and ankylosis. Arch. Oral Biol., *18*:1021–1040, 1973.

Parker, W. S., Frisbe, H. E., and Grant, T. S.: The experimental production of dental ankylosis. Angle Orthod., *34*:103, 1964.

Rule, J. T., Zacherl, W. A., and Pfefferle, A. M.: The relationship between ankylosed molars and multiple enamel defects. J. Dent. Child., *39*:29–35, 1972.

Rygh, P., and Reitan, K.: Changes in the supporting tissues of submerged deciduous molars with and without permanent successors. Odont. Tskr., *72*:345, 1964.

Sharway, A. M., Mills, P. B., and Gibbons, R.: Multiple ankylosis occurring in rat teeth. Oral Surg., *26*:896–860, 1968.

Shaw, J., and Samuels, H. S.: The "submerged" tooth. Oral Surg., *14*:440–441, 1961.

Via, W. F.: Submerged deciduous molars: familial tendencies. J.A.D.A., *69*:127–129, 1964.

Agenesis

Baum, B. J., and Cohen, M. M.: Studies on agenesis in the permanent dentition. Am. J. Phys. Anthrop., *35*:125–128, 1971*a*.

Baum, B. J., and Cohen, M. M.: Patterns of size reduction in hypodontia. J. Dent. Res., *50*:779, 1971*b*.

Baum, B. J., and Cohen, M. M.: Agenesis and tooth size in the permanent dentition. Angle Orthod., *41*:100–102, 1971*c*.

Baum, B. J., and Cohen, M. M.: Decreased odontometric sex differences in individuals with dental agenesis. Am. J. Phys. Anthrop., *38*:739–742, 1973.

Brown, R. V.: The pattern and frequency of congenitally absent teeth. Iowa Dent. J., *45*:60–61, 1957.

Clayton, J. M.: Congenital dental anomalies occurring in 557 children. J. Dent. Child., *23*:206–208, 1956.

Glenn, F. B.: Incidence of congenitally missing permanent teeth in a private pedodontic practice. J. Dent. Child., *28*:317–321, 1961.

Glenn, F. B.: A consecutive six year study on the prevalence of congenitally missing teeth in private pedodontic practice of two geographically separated areas. J. Dent. Child., *31*:264–270, 1964.

Grahnen, H.: Hypodontia in the permanent dentition, a clinical and genetic investigation. Dent. Abs., *2*:308–309, 1956.

Keene, H. J.: The relationship between third molar agensis and the morphologic variants of molar teeth. Angle Orthod., *35*:289–298, 1965.

Muller, T. J., Hill, I. N., Peterson, A. C., and Blayney, J. R.: A survey of congenitally missing permanent teeth. J.A.D.A., *81*:101–107, 1970.

Valinotti, J. R.: The congenitally absent premolar problem. Angle Orthod., *28*:36–45, 1958.

Werther, R., and Rothenberg, F.: Anodontia: A review of its etiology with presentation of a case. Am. J. Orthod., *25*:61–81, 1939.

Treatment for Mandibular Incisor Crowding

Dominik, K.: Vertical grinding of teeth in jaw orthopedics. Czasopismo Stomatologiczne, *25*:187–192, 1972.

Hudson, A. L.: A study of the effects of mesiodistal reduction of mandibular anterior teeth. Am. J. Orthod., *42*:615–624, 1956.

Paskow, H.: Self-alignment following interproximal stripping. Am. J. Orthod., *58*:240–249, 1970.

Peck, H., and Peck, S.: An index for assessing tooth shape deviations as applied to the mandibular incisors. Am. J. Orthod., *61*:384–401, 1972.

Peck, S., and Peck, H.: Orthodontic aspects of dental anthropology. Angle Orthod., *45*:92–102, 1975.

Peck, H., and Peck, S.: Reproximation (enamel stripping) as an essential orthodontic treatment ingredient. Transactions of Third International Orthodontic Congress, pp. 513–523. Crosby Lockwood Staples, 1975.

Tabori, P., and Vidovic, Z.: Trimming of teeth as a therapeutic method in orthodontics. Stomatololoski Glasnik Sribje (Beograd), *17*:189–196, 1970.

Suggested Readings

This book was written to make the practitioner aware of minor occlusal disharmonies and their early treatment for the prevention of major occlusal disharmonies. The text is practical in nature and it is the hope of the author that the suggested references will help the practitioner toward a better understanding of growth and development and of the multifactorial etiological entities that play a role in the development of occlusal disharmonies in the primary and early mixed permanent dentitions.

Texts

Adams, C. P.: The Design and Construction of Removable Orthodontic Appliances. Bristol, England, John Wright and Sons, Ltd., 1957.

Adams, C. P.: The Design and Construction of Removable Appliances. 4th Ed. Baltimore, Williams & Wilkins, 1970.

Anderson, G. M.: Practical Orthodontics. St. Louis, C. V. Mosby Co., 9th Ed., 1966.

Barnett, E. M.: Pediatric Occlusal Therapy. St. Louis, C. V. Mosby Co., 1974.

Begg, P. R., and Kesling, P. C.: Begg Orthodontic Theory and Technique. 2nd Ed. Philadelphia, W. B. Saunders Co., 1965.

Beresford, J. S.: Orthodontic Diagnosis. Bristol, England, John Wright and Sons, Ltd., 1965.

Berke, J. S.: The Linked Arch Appliance. New York, Charles Press, 1957.

Dickson, G. C.: Orthodontics in General Dental Practice. London, Pitman Medical Publishing Co., Ltd., 1959.

Dickson, G. C.: Orthodontics in General Dental Practice. Philadelphia, Lea & Febiger, 1964.

Dickson, G. C.: An Atlas of Removable Orthodontic Appliances. London, Pitman Medical Publishing Co., Ltd., 1965.

Finn, S. B.: Clinical Pedodontics. 4th Ed. Philadelphia, W. B. Saunders Co., 1973.

Fischer, B.: Clinical Orthodontics, A Guide to the Sectional Method. Philadelphia, W. B. Saunders Co., 1957.

Forde, T. H.: The Principles and Practice of Oral Dynamics. New York, Exposition Press, 1964.

Geoffrion, P.: Clinical Application of the Twin-Wire Mechanism. Paris, Julien Prelat, 1962.

Graber, T. M.: Orthodontics: Principles and Practice. 3rd Ed. Philadelphia, W. B. Saunders Co., 1972.

Graber, T. M., and Swain, B. F. (Eds.): Current Orthodontic Concepts and Techniques. 2nd Ed. Philadelphia, W. B. Saunders Co., 1975.

Harvold, E. P.: The Activator in Interceptive Orthodontics. St. Louis, C. V. Mosby Co., 1974.

Hirshfeld, L.: Minor Tooth Movement in General Practice. St. Louis, C. V. Mosby Co., 1966.

Jarabak, J. R.: Technique and Treatment with Light-Wire Edgewise Appliance. St. Louis, C. V. Mosby Co., 1972.

Law, D. B., Lewis, T. M., and Davis, J. M.: An Atlas of Pedodontics. Philadelphia, W. B. Saunders Co., 1969.

Lindstrom, A.: Introduction to Orthodontics. New York, McGraw-Hill Book Co., Inc., 1960.

McDonald, R. E.: Pedodontics. Vol 1: Management of Space Maintenance Problems. Vol. 2: Diagnosis and Correction of Minor Irregularities in the Developing Dentition. St. Louis, C. V. Mosby Co., 1963.

McDonald, R. E.: Dentistry for the Child and Adolescent. St. Louis, C. V. Mosby Co., 1969.

Moyers, R. E.: Handbook of Orthodontics for the Student and General Practitioner. 3rd Ed. Chicago, Year Book Medical Publishers, 1973.

Saltzmann, J. A.: Orthodontics: Principles and Prevention. Philadelphia, J. B. Lippincott Co., 1957.

Sassouni, V.: The Face in Five Dimensions. Morgantown, West Virginia, School of Dentistry, West Virginia University, 1962.

Sassouni, V., and Forest, E. J.: Orthodontics in Dental Practices. St. Louis, C. V. Mosby Co., 1971.

Schwartz, A. M., and Gratzinger, M.: Removable Orthodontic Appliances. Philadelphia, W. B. Saunders Co., 1960.

Tarpley, B. W.: Technique and Treatment with the Labio-Lingual Appliance. St. Louis, C. V. Mosby Co., 1961.

Thurow, R.: Technique and Treatment with the Edgewise Appliance. St. Louis, C. V. Mosby Co., 1962.

Thurow, R.: Edgewise Orthodontics. Technique and Treatment with Edgewise Appliance. St. Louis, C. V. Mosby Co., 1966.

Thurow, R.: Atlas of Orthodontic Principles. St. Louis, C. V. Mosby Co., 1970.

Tulley, W. J., and Campbell, A. C.: A Manual of Practical Orthodontics. Bristol, England, John Wright and Sons, Ltd., 1970.

Tulley, W. J., and Cyer, B. S.: Orthodontics-Treatment for the Adult. Bristol, England, John Wright and Sons, Ltd., 1967.

White, T. C., Gardner, J. H., and Leighton, B. C.: Orthodontics for Dental Students. London, Staples Press, 1954.

White, T. C., Gardner, J. H., and Leighton, B. C.: Orthodontics. London, Staples Press, 1967.

Wilbrecht, A. T.: Crozat Appliances in Interceptive Maxillofacial Orthopedics. Published for the Wiebrecht Foundation by Schmidt, Milwaukee, 1969.

Growth and Development

Cohen, M. M.: Clinical studies in the development of the dental height. Am. J. Orthod., *36*:917–932, 1950.

Cohen, M. M., and Garn, S. M.: Factors in occlusion. Am. J. Orthod., *40*:671–685, 1954.

Fanning, E. A.: A longitudinal study of tooth formation and root resorption. N.Z. Dent. J., *57*:202–217, 1961.

Fanning, E. A.: Effect of extraction of deciduous molars on the formation and eruption of their successors. Angle Orthod., *32*:44–53, 1962.

Frolich, F. J.: A longitudinal study of untreated Class II type malocclusions. Trans. Europ. Orthod., Soc., 1961.

Horowitz, S. L., Converse, J. K., and Gerstman, L. J.: Craniofacial relationships in mandibular prognathism. Arch. Oral Bio., *14*:121–131, 1969.

Hurme, V. O.: Ranges of normalcy in the eruption of permanent teeth. J. Dent. Child., 1949.

MacLaughlin, J. A., Fogels, H. R., and Shiere, F. R.: The influence of premature primary molar extraction on bicuspid eruption. J. Dent. Child., *34*:399–405, 1967.

Moorrees, C. F. A., Gron, A., Lebret, L., Yen, P., and Frolich, F.: Growth studies of the dentition. Am. J. Orthod., *55*:600–616, 1969.

Moorrees, C. F. A., Thomsen, S. Ø., Jensen, E., and Yen, P. K. J.: Mesiodistal crown diameters of the deciduous and permanent teeth in individuals. J. Dent. Res., *36*:39–47, 1957.

Shiere, F. R., and Frankl, S. N.: The effect of deciduous tooth infection on permanent teeth. Dent. Prog., *2*:59–64, 1961.

Van der Linden, F. D. G. M.: Genetic and environmental factors in dentofacial morphology. Am. J. Orthod., *52*:576–583, 1966.

Serial Extractions

Carr, L. M.: The effect of extraction of deciduous molars on the eruption of bicuspid teeth. Aust. Dent. J., *8*:130–136, 1963.

Dewel, B. F.: Clinical observations on the axial inclination of teeth. Am. J. Orthod., *35*:98–115, 1949.

Dewel, B. F.: Serial extraction in orthodontics: Indications, objectives, and treatment procedures. Am. J. Orthod., *40*:906–926, 1954.

Dewel, B. F.: The indications and technique of the edgewise appliance in serial extraction procedures. Trans. Europ. Orthod. Soc., pp. 84–107, 1956.

Dewel, B. F.: A critical analysis of serial extraction in orthodontic treatment. Am. J. Orthod., *45*:424–455, 1959.

Dewel, B. F.: Objectives of mixed dentition treatment in orthodontics. Am. J. Orthod., *50*:504–520, 1964.

Dewel, B. F.: Serial extraction: Its limitations and contraindications in orthodontic treatment. Am. J. Orthod., *53*:904–921, 1967.

Dewel, B. F.: Prerequisites in serial extraction. Am. J. Orthod., *55*:633–639, 1969.

Graber, T. M.: Serial extraction: A continuous diagnostic and decisional process. Am. J. Orthod., *60*:541–575, 1971.

Heath, J.: The interception of malocclusion by planned serial extraction. N.Z. Dent. J., *49*:77–88, 1953.

Hotz, R.: Zur Fage der Zahnevtraktionen in der Behandlung von Zahnstellungsano-malien. Schweiz. Monatsschr. Zahn., *50*:1940.

Hotz, R.: Active supervision of the erupted teeth by extraction. Trans. Europ. Orthod. Soc., pp. 34–47, 1947, 1948.

Hotz, R. P.: Guidance of eruption versus serial extraction. Am. J. Orthod., *58*:1–20, 1970.

Kjellgren, B.: Serial extraction as a corrective procedure in dental orthopedic therapy. Trans. Europ. Orthod. Soc., pp. 134–160, 1947, 1948.

Maj, G.: Serial extraction in Class I mixed dentition cases. Am. J. Orthod., *57*:393–399, 1970.

Mayne, W. R.: Serial extraction. *In* Graber, T. M.: Current Orthodontic Concepts and Techniques. Vol. I. 2nd Ed. Philadelphia, W. B. Saunders Co., 1975.

Profit, W. R., and Bennett, I. C.: Space maintenance, serial extraction and the general practitioner. J.A.D.A., *74*:411–419, 1967.

Ringenberg, Q. M.: Influence of serial extraction on growth and development of the maxilla and mandible. Am. J. Orthod., *53*:19–26, 1967.

Sanin, C., Nakamura, S., and Savar, B. S.: Serial extraction without orthodontic treatment. J.A.D.A., *81*:653–661, 1970.

Taylor, R. F.: Controlled serial extraction. Am. J. Orthod., *60*:576–599, 1971.

Epidemiology

Ast, D. B., Carlos, J. P., and Cons, J. C.: The prevalence and characteristics of malocclusion among senior high school students in upstate New York. Am. J. Orthod., *51*:437–445, 1965.

Gardiner, J. H.: A survey of malocclusion and some aetiological factors in 1000 Sheffield school children. Dent. Pract., *6*:187–201, 1956.

Helms, S.: Malocclusion in Danish children with adolescent dentitions: An epidemiological study. Am. J. Orthod., *54*:352–366, 1968.

Massler, M., and Frankel, J. M.: Prevalence of malocclusion in children aged 14 to 18 years. Am. J. Orthod., *37*:751–768, 1951.

Mills, L. F.: Epidemiologic studies of occlusion. IV. The prevalence of malocclusion in a population of 1455 school children. J. Dent. Res., *45*:332–336, 1966.

Newman, G. V.: Prevalence of malocclusion in children six to fourteen years of age and treatment in preventable cases. J.A.D.A., *52*:566–575, 1956.

Worms, F. W., Meskin, L. H., and Isaacson, R. J.: Open-bite. Am. J. Orthod., *59*:589–595, 1971.

Treatment

Abrams, I. N.: Oral muscle pressures. Angle Orthod., *33*:83–104, 1963.

Bernstein, L.: The ACCO appliance. J. Pract. Orthod., *3*:461–468, 1969.

Bernstein, L.: Treatment of Class II, division 1. Maximum anchorage cases with the ACCO appliance. J. Clin. Orthod., *4*:1970.

Cheney, E. A.: Treatment planning and therapy in the mixed dentition. Am. J. Orthod., *49*:568–580, 1963.

Denholtz, M.: A method of harnessing lip pressure to move teeth. J. Amer. Soc. Study Orthod., December 1963.

Denholtz, M.: An effective procedure to help guide the developing dentition into proper occlusion. J. Dent. Child., *31*:192–197, 1964.

Denholtz, M.: A method for recontouring lips into a more esthetic appearance. Int. J. Orthod., *3*:5–10, 1965.

Dewel, B. F.: Objectives of mixed dentition treatment in orthodontics. Am. J. Orthod., *50*:504–520, 1964.

Haas, A. J.: Palatal expansion: Just the beginning of dentofacial orthopedics. Am. J. Orthod., *57*:219–255, 1970.

Harvold, E.: Some biological aspects of orthodontic treatment in the transitional dentition. Am. J. Orthod., *49*:1–14, 1963.

King, F. W.: Looking back: The lessons of fifteen years of mixed dentition treatment. Am. J. Orthod., *54*:733–748, 1968.

Kloehn, S. J.: A new approach to analysis and treatment in mixed dentition. Am. J. Orthod., *39*:161–186, 1953.

Levitas, T. C.: Examine the habit—evaluate the treatment. J. Dent. Child., *37*:34, 1970.

Massler, Maury, and Chopra, B.: The palatal crib for the correction of oral habits. J. Dent. Child., 1950.

Murillo, J. C.: Mixed dentition treatment with the selective functional appliance. Am. J. Orthod., *63*:596–605, 1973.

Murray, R. B.: Treatment planning and therapy in the mixed dentition. Am. J. Orthod., *49*:641–657, 1963.

Ruff, R. M.: Orthodontic treatment in the mixed dentition. Am. J. Orthod., *57*:502–518, 1970.

Sather, A. H., Mayfield, S. B., and Nelson, D. H.: Effects of muscular anchorage appliances on deficient mandibular arch length. Am. J. Orthod., *60*:68–78, 1971.

Van der Linden, F. D. G. M.: The application of removable orthodontic appliances in multi-band techniques. Angle Orthod., *39*:114–117, 1969.

Van der Linden, F. D. G. M.: The removable orthodontic appliance. Am. J. Orthod., *59*:376–385, 1971.

Zwemer, T. J.: Ten rules of the mixed dentition. J. Dent. Child., *35*:298–304, 1968.

Prosthesis

Chuchmai, L. D.: Replacement of lost teeth and its role in preventing malformation of teeth and jaws. Stomatologia, *48*:65–68, 1969.

Lindahl, R. L.: Denture techniques suitable for growing arches. Dent. Clin. N. Am., pp. 649–660, November, 1961.

Voss, R.: The possibilities and limitations of prosthetic replacement of missing incisors in the young patient. Fortschr. Kieferorthop., *30*:89–101, 1969.

INDEX

Page numbers in *italics* refer to illustrations; (t) indicates tables.